QUICK
& EASY

energy
boosters

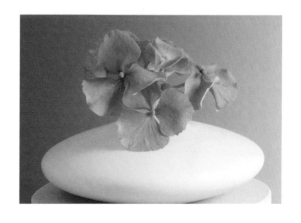

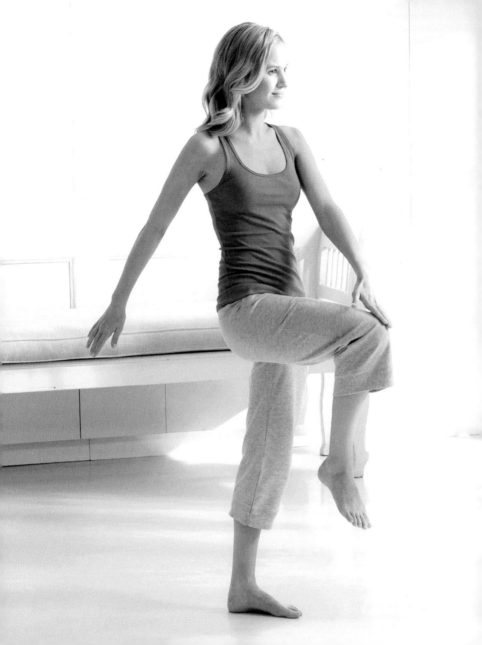

DUNCAN BAIRD PUBLISHERS

LONDON

QUICK & EASY

energy boosters

Janet Wright

5-minute routines for

anyone

anytime

anywhere

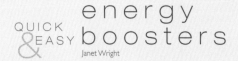

energy
QUICK & EASY boosters

Janet Wright

First published in the United Kingdom and Ireland in 2009 by
Duncan Baird Publishers Ltd
Sixth Floor
Castle House
75–76 Wells Street
London WIT 3QH

Conceived, created and designed by Duncan Baird Publishers

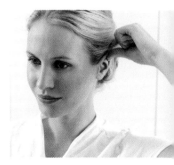

Managing Editor: Grace Cheetham
Editor: Katey Mackenzie
Managing Designer: Manisha Patel
Designer: Jantje Doughty
Commissioned photography: Jules Selmes

British Library Cataloguing-in-Publication Data:
A CIP record for this book is available from the British Library

ISBN: 978-1-84483-784-7

10 9 8 7 6 5 4 3

Typeset in Gill Sans, Nofret and Helvetica Neue
Colour reproduction by Scanhouse, Malaysia
Printed in China by Imago

To Cora and Richard Kemball–Cook,
genial hosts whose generosity extends
way beyond the call of friendship.
Thanks for all your support, including
allowing people time and space to
revive in the tranquil atmosphere
you create around you.

To everyone who has taught me the
techniques used in this book. Especially
to Cora, who motivates me by being
living proof of yoga's effectiveness.

And to David Hall for everything.

contents

introduction

There's no real mystery or magic surrounding how energized you feel. At the most basic level, your body creates energy when it metabolizes food – which is why your diet is so important when it comes to how much get up and go you have. However, in order for the internal combustion process to take place, your body needs a catalyst – and that catalyst is oxygen. Breathing and circulation are fundamental for maximizing the supply of oxygen to your body's tissues to create energy; while muscles that are free from tension and a body that moves easily and effortlessly use oxygen more efficiently, liberate trapped energy and generally help to make you feel more upbeat. In addition, if you can make use of the feel-good hormones that the brain releases when you exercise, you will feel more energized because you feel more positive.

concepts of energy

The physiological view of the body's energy is only one way to look at things. In Eastern thought, from China and Japan to Tibet and India, the physical body is underpinned by an energetic, or "subtle", body. This subtle body is made up of a system of energy channels, sometimes called meridians, through which vital energy or life force flows. This energy is known as *chi* in China, *ki* in Japan and *prana* in India. In China and Japan, the seat of all energy is the body's *hara* or "sea of vitality".

In all Eastern belief systems, when the flow of energy is blocked or sluggish, ill health results. To combat this, Eastern practices provide myriad ways to increase energy-flow through the body or to remove obstructions to it. For example, the Japanese practice of shiatsu aims to maintain the free flow of energy by pressing on key points around the body; the Chinese practice of chi gung controls energy-flow through the co-ordination of breath and movement; and, in the Indian practice of yoga, postural exercises and breath control release and optimize the flow of energy around the subtle body. These and other techniques, including Western practices, are introduced on pages 10–15.

the main energy blockers

There are several lifestyle factors that, in Western terms, sap physical energy and in Eastern thought block the flow of subtle energy. Either way, the results are tiredness, lethargy and ill health.

• **Stress** Nothing depletes your energy more than stress. An almost inevitable by-product of modern living, stress causes tension in the muscles, which in turn restricts the body's circulation, reducing the amount of oxygen available for the metabolism to work effectively. The effort of moving when you're using tired, tightened muscles saps energy, too. But, of course, stress is not only a physical affliction.

7

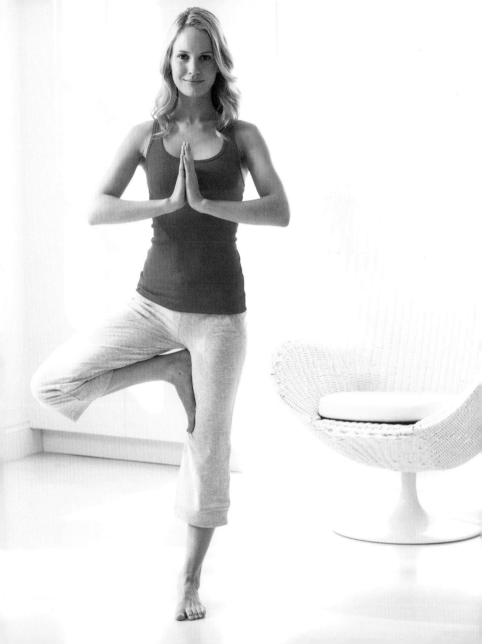

Mental stress soaks up your body's energy in industrial quantities. Meanwhile, useful energy is diverted away from healthy activities, such as metabolizing your food or expelling toxins, to dealing with all the thought patterns associated with anxiety and fear. Your body prepares itself to deal with stress defensively by diverting energy to the muscles to enable the "fight-or-flight" response. When it does this repeatedly, as during prolonged periods of stress, without active efforts to put a stop to the process, you may become lethargic, and even ill. Many of the stress-busting exercises in this book (such as In Your Bathroom on pages 48–9) are intended to restore a state of deep calm, washing away anxiety and leaving you feeling lighter and more energized. Others, such as Vitality Enhancer (pages 92–3), which derives from shiatsu, aims to work directly on the flow of energy through your subtle body to restore balance.

• **Poor sleep patterns** Studies show that many of us are spending increasingly less time asleep, giving the body less time to restore and replenish. All the exercises in this book will help you to sleep better by improving your physical well-being, thus relieving aches and pains that may disturb sleep, or by clearing mental clutter.

• **Poor nutrition** As I said right at the beginning, what you eat is fundamental to your levels of energy. A diet that is high in processed

9

foods will deplete your energy, whereas one that is packed with fresh fruits and vegetables, healthy carbohydrates such as whole grains and wholewheat bread, and high-protein foods such as poultry, fish and tofu is energy-giving. However, eating the right foods is no help if your digestion is poor, so there's a Lunchtime Balancer on pages 28–9 that will help you to slow down and digest essential nutrients – feel free to use it after any meal of the day.

• **Lack of exercise** Rather like the adage that you have to spend money to make money, sometimes you have to expend energy to feel more energetic. Regular exercise speeds your metabolism, improves your stamina (reducing the risk of injury, as well as making you physically stronger), and keeps your everyday energy levels high. Many of the exercises in this book will energize you through movement.

energy-boosting practices

As with most things in life, nothing comes from nothing and we need to make a little effort to improve our levels of energy. However, that effort needn't be a chore nor difficult nor time-consuming. This book is packed with dozens of "five-minute miracles" that will give you quick, healthy energy boosts when you most need them. All of the exercises are drawn from popular energizing techniques from both the East and the West. Used together, they provide an arsenal of approaches that will lead you to health and vitality.

• **Aerobic exercise** Simple and effective, aerobic exercise would cost a fortune if someone could bottle and sell it! Any exercise that makes your heart beat faster and lets you work up a bit of a sweat is aerobic and will stimulate your body's production of feel-good hormones, improve your circulation, and boost your stamina. Brisk walking, swimming, running and dancing are all good forms of aerobic exercise, as are several of the exercises in chapters 3 and 4. Take care, though – don't work yourself so hard that you become completely out of breath, you should still be able to speak.

• **Breath control** Dedicating some time to regulating your breath not only increases the amount of oxygen you use effectively, but also provides a quick-fix solution for stress, calming your mind and restoring a soothing sense of equilibrium. This, in turn, reduces your body's stress response (see page 9). Exercises such as Stress Reliever on pages 102–3 are perfect for this.

• **Chi gung and tai chi** Translating literally as "energy work", chi gung derives from Chinese martial arts. It co-ordinates breath and movement to release blocked energy in the meridians and harmonize the mind and body for overall well-being. The martial art tai chi has

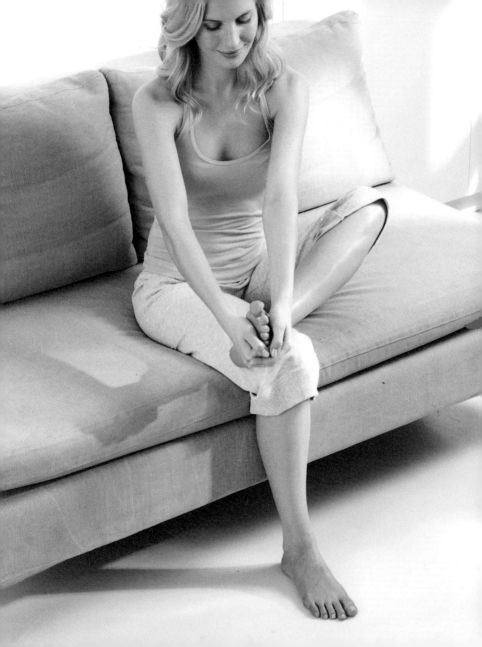

been proven to boost circulation, regulate breathing and lower stress and in all these ways it will help to boost your body's energy levels.

- **Meditation and visualization** Almost all ancient Eastern practices include some form of meditation or visualization. Central to Eastern belief is the idea that the body and mind are inextricably linked and that the vitality of one will affect the vitality of the other. Learning to meditate, and practising every day, harnesses core mental energy and helps to shift psychological blockage that may prevent you from living life to the full. Learning to declutter your mind through meditation and visualization (for example, see the Mental Refresher on pages 90–1) will rein in any runaway mental processes, making you feel happier and more in control of your life. With a positive mental attitude and positive emotions come improved energy levels.

- **Yoga** The use of postures to free up energy and improve strength and stamina is known as Hatha yoga and originated in India many centuries ago. Some yoga practices encourage stillness in a posture (such as the Lunchtime Balancer on pages 28–9), while some encourage movement through a series or sequence of postures (such as the Chest Opener on pages 112–3). The aim should always be to co-ordinate your breath with your movement and to practise the postures in a controlled, calm way.

• **Shiatsu** This form of Japanese massage is said to stimulate energy points (acupressure points) in the body using finger pressure, thus balancing the flow of energy through the meridians to improve well-being. The practice is simple and highly effective. Many of the exercises in this book are derived from shiatsu and some are combined with reflexology (see below) for maximum benefits.

• **Reflexology** Developed in the 20th century in the USA (although thought to originate thousands of years ago), reflexology – also known as zone therapy – is a practice using certain pressure points on the feet or hands to correspond to particular parts of the body. Stimulating these pressure points is meant to address any energy imbalances in the corresponding body part. Also included are reflexology exercises that aim to work on the pineal gland (which regulates the body's sleep-wake patterns), as well as points said to improve brain activity and the functioning of the internal organs that regulate the balance of energy through the body.

• **Massage** All forms of massage will improve circulation in the body and several techniques are included in the book. Body brushing helps to stimulate the flow of lymph around the body, which improves immunity and the elimination of toxins. Hydrotherapy massage, using the warm water of a shower (see Shower Time on pages 24–5), is a wonderful way to start the day, easing tension out of the muscles and lifting the spirits. Ayurvedic massage stimulates the body's own healing energies to promote vitality. If you are massaging a partner, note that some massages (such as the Back Massager on pages 116–7) don't need oil and can be performed with the person fully clothed.

Although all of the exercises in this book can provide individual quick fixes, I urge you also to look at the sequences set out on pages 124–5. Longer sessions that combine techniques will naturally give longer-lasting benefits. In addition, movement techniques, such as yoga, tai chi and chi gung, will be most fruitful if you back up daily sessions at home by going to weekly or twice-weekly classes with a qualified teacher. All the practices in the book are governed by professional, bodies that will have a list of registered teachers in your area.

other ways to boost your energy

It's important to supplement your physical and mental efforts to boost your energy with some simple lifestyle changes. For example, have a look around you and pinpoint areas of clutter in your home and then have a declutter day – clearing your outer space is just as important as clearing your inner space. Simplify your life as much

15

as possible. For example, if you have children, rather than running from one activity to the next with them, schedule some time just to have fun together. Having fun is one of the most energizing activities of all. Get your shopping delivered, pay the bills by standing order, order a healthy take-away once a week. There are myriad small ways to conserve your energy – and when combined, the resulting positive effects on your overall zest for life can be huge.

contraindications

Although the exercises in this book are suitable for most people and all age groups, don't push your body beyond its limits. Check with your doctor before you embark on any new exercises if you have a known health condition and do not do anything that could conflict with your doctor's advice. If you experience pain, stop the exercise at once, and see your doctor if it persists. Keep breathing naturally; only one exercise (Anxiety Settler on pages 100–1) requires you to hold your breath for a short time, but avoid this if you have high blood pressure.

Finally, if you are unusually tired without any obvious reason, see your doctor. Chronic lethargy could be a warning sign for a number of health conditions, which can be successfully treated if diagnosed at an early stage. Never ignore your body.

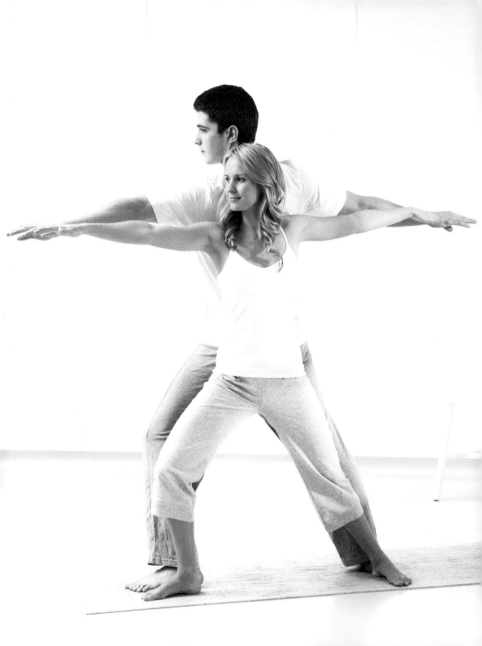

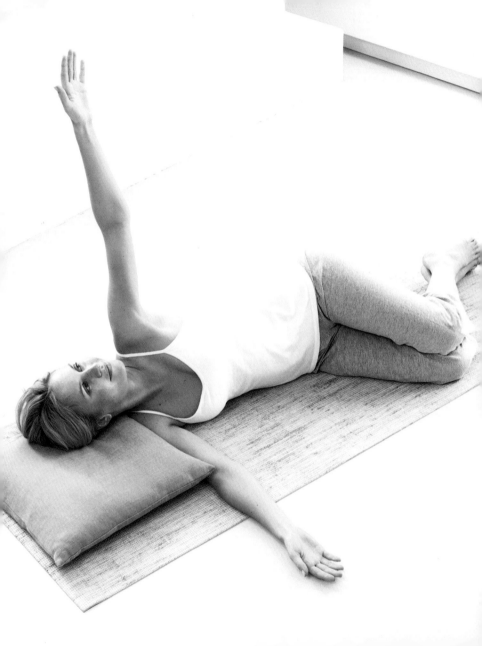

how to use this book

The chapters in this book have been designed to give you every opportunity to harmonize your energy whenever you need to. In Chapter 1 the exercises focus on particular times of the day – for example, a boost for the morning, something to restore energy in the mid-afternoon and calming exercises to make sure that your sleep is as restful as possible. Chapter 2 shows you that you don't need to have a special place in which to boost your energy – anywhere will do. I've something to add to this, too – practise outside whenever you can. Numerous studies show that people are healthier, happier, more energetic and better able to cope when they are able to spend time among greenery and feel closer to nature. Chapters 3 and 4 look at boosting physical and mental energy respectively with tailored techniques; while Chapter 5 offers ideas for practising with a partner. The book ends with several sequences that combine the exercises in the rest of the book. They are wonderful for a longer practice.

When you are full of energy, your skin glows and you feel on top of the world. Even the tasks that once seemed daunting are suddenly effortless and fun. It is my wish that this book will show you how to boost your mental and physical energy, so that it flows into every aspect of your life giving you the vitality to enjoy living to the full.

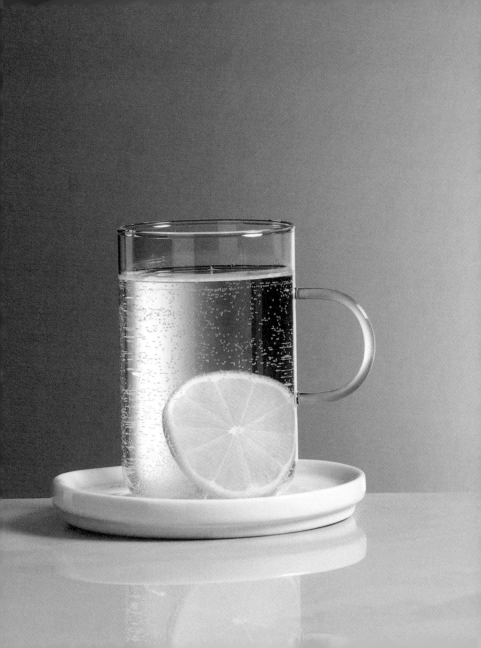

anytime

Whether it's first thing in the morning to prepare you for the day,

to refresh you during a mid-afternoon energy slump, to boost your

mind-power for a meeting, or to invigorate you for a night out,

five minutes can be all you need to top up your energy levels at any

time of day, or to balance and calm them for a restful night.

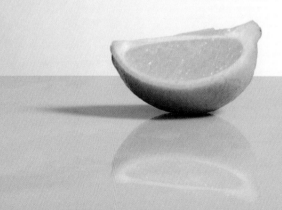

morning stretch awakening

start the day well with energy-harnessing stretches

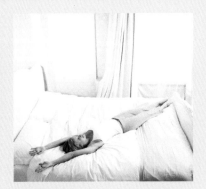 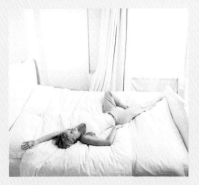

1 Getting up soon after you wake allows you to use your morning energy, which drains away if you stay in bed for more than a few minutes. Lie on your back with your eyes shut as you move gently into wakefulness. Then slowly lift your arms above your head, breathe in and stretch from the tips of your fingers to your toes.

2 Breathe out and relax. Breathe in, and stretch your right hand and right foot away from each other, then breathe out as you relax. Continue breathing in time with your movements as you stretch your left arm and left leg. Next, stretch your left arm and your right leg, then your right arm and your left leg. Breathe normally throughout.

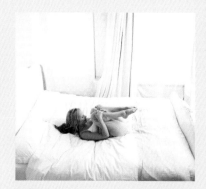
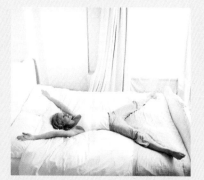

3 When you have gently stretched your arms and legs, and both sides of your body, bring your knees up and in toward your chest. Hug your knees close and curl your body into a ball, bringing your forehead up toward your knees. Feel the gentle stretch along your back muscles, without putting any strain on your lower spine.

4 On an inbreath, stretch out strongly to the tips of your fingers and toes, arms and legs apart, making a powerful and expansive star shape. Bring your knees back in to your chest, then do the star stretch again. Starting the day with this set of rhythmic stretches brings you smoothly to full consciousness without feeling rushed.

23

1 A morning shower is a pleasant way of mentally getting into daytime gear. Don't rush it, but make the most of its energizing potential as a form of hydrotherapy. Before you begin to wash, start by being fully present in the moment, enjoying the feel of the warm water as it flows over your body.

2 As you rinse off the soapy water, raise your right arm and watch the water flowing down it. Do the same with your left arm. The refreshing qualities of a shower are more than just physical: the touch and sound of breaking water will lift your spirits and increase feelings of vitality – washing away your sleepiness.

3 Take the shower head out of its holder, if this is possible, and direct the flow over your face and body, visualizing it washing away the old stale energy. Run it down your back, and over your hips and legs. Reduce the temperature, then alternate between cool and warm water.

4 Finally, turn the temperature down and let the cool water flow over your face and neck. Work your way up to setting the shower fully to cold for the last few minutes, if you can. You'll find that you'll step out tingling with vitality. Finish by briskly towelling yourself dry.

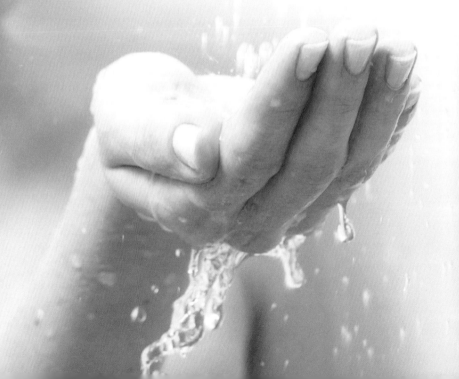

shower
time
refreshing

splash the last traces of sleepiness
away with hydrotherapy

1 Stand at the foot of the stairs. Step up onto the bottom step with your left foot, and bring your right foot up to join it, putting your heels down each time. You can rest your hand on the wall, if needed, but do not to lean on it as your weight should be squarely over your feet.

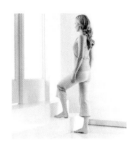

2 Step down with the left foot, then the right. Repeat, starting on the right: right foot up, left foot up, right foot down, left foot down. Repeat this sequence at least 12 times, being careful to put your whole foot down each time, not stepping up and down on your toes.

3 Standing on the bottom step, check that your back is in a neutral position – neither slumped nor arched – and hold in your abdominal muscles firmly to support your spine. Still holding the wall, move back until only your toes and the balls of your feet are on the step.

4 *(right)* Lower your heels and hold the stretch for up to 10 seconds. Bring your heels close together and repeat the calf stretch with your toes turned out. Then bring your toes close together and do the same again with heels turned out. Do each stretch three to six times.

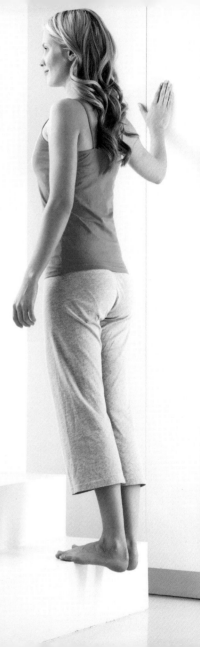

mid-morning
activator
stimulating

use your morning break to
boost your circulation

1 Walk mindfully to a quiet place. With the weight on your right leg, lift your left heel as you breathe in. Bring your left foot smoothly forward and place it on the floor as you breathe out, letting your weight move onto your left leg. Continue breathing at your normal rate and taking one step per breath.

2 When you reach a spot where you won't be interrupted, stand with your feet close together, arms by your sides. Continue breathing in the same steady, relaxed rhythm. Rock slightly on your feet until you feel your body weight centred between your toes and your heels, and also between your left and right sides.

3 *(right)* Move your weight onto your left foot and bring your right heel off the ground. Swivel on the ball of your right foot so that your sole is against your left ankle. Turn your right knee out. Bring your right foot up against your left calf or thigh. Hold your hands in front of your chest, palms together, in a prayer position.

4 To help keep your balance, focus on something static a short distance in front of you. Keep breathing steadily and hold the pose for five breaths. If you start to really wobble, put your right foot down and stand with your toes on the floor and your right sole against your left ankle. Repeat on the other side.

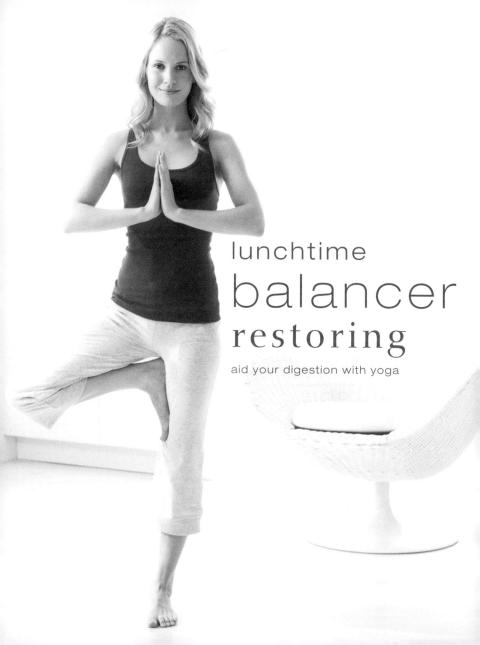

lunchtime
balancer
restoring

aid your digestion with yoga

afternoon wake-up reinvigorating

leap out of a tea-time energy slump

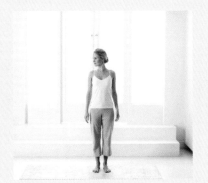

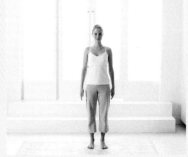

1 Stand up tall. Using very small movements, rock slightly forward onto your toes and then back again onto your heels. Explore the feeling of your soles against the floor. Tip your weight to the left and right sides of your feet and come to a central position. Turn your head to look round from side to side and then up and down.

2 Bring your head to rest in a central position. Allow your shoulders to relax, with your arms hanging loosely by your sides. Stand with your legs straight and strong, engaging your thigh muscles as if lifting your kneecaps upward. Keep your feet well rooted to the floor. Hold this stance for 10 deep, steady breaths.

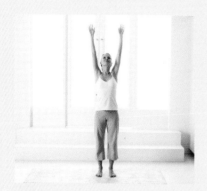

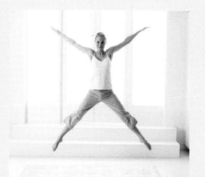

3 Raise your arms above your head and lean back from the waist, looking up. Don't let your head fall back and keep your neck long. To avoid hurting your lower back, engage your abdominal muscles. Don't let your pelvis slip forward or arch your back. Feel your legs holding you strong and steady as your arms reach up.

4 Breathe in as you stretch up, then breathe out and bring your arms down by your sides. On your next in-breath, leap up with arms and legs wide. Land with your knees bent, bringing your heels down as well as your toes. Repeat this three times, feeling the energy coursing through your body to the tips of your fingers and toes.

1 Just before you go to bed, find somewhere quiet and peaceful to sit down. For best results sit with your back straight and supported – a dining chair would be ideal – and your feet flat on the floor. Feel your breathing slow down naturally and allow any stray thoughts that wander into your mind to simply float away.

2 *(right)* Close your eyes to let your sense of touch take over. Rest one thumb on your temple. Using one finger, lightly explore the area between your eyebrows and just above, until you find a natural dip. Gently massage this for a minute to help soothe racing thoughts.

3 Rest one ankle on your lap and cup it in the other hand, so that you're touching the small bones that protrude on the inside and outside of the heel. Just below the bone on the inside of the heel is an acupressure point which, when pressed, can help to prepare you for sleep.

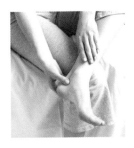

4 Just behind the bone on the outside of your heel you'll find another relaxing acupressure point. Together, these two points can promote healthy sleep, even for people suffering from insomnia. Press gently with your thumb and massage around the whole area using a small circular motion. Repeat on your other foot.

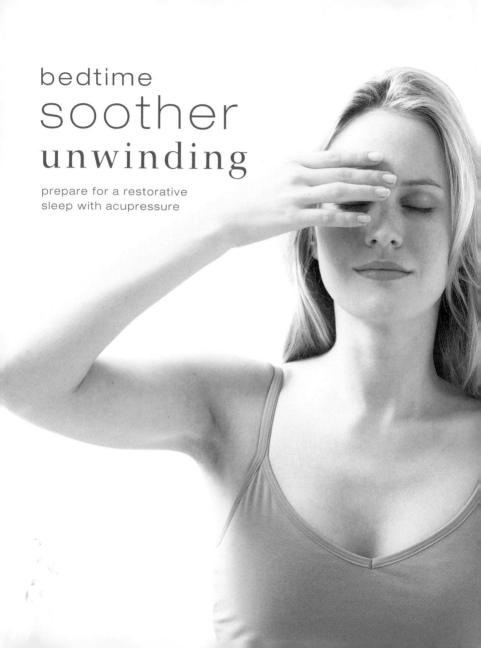

bedtime
soother
unwinding

prepare for a restorative
sleep with acupressure

weekend moves
balancing

clear away stale energy from your working week with chi gung

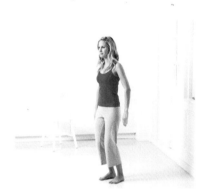

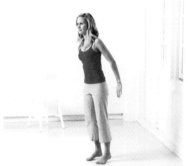

1 Stand with your feet about hip-width apart, knees very slightly bent, feeling well grounded. Stand up straight, but without arching your back: let your spine find its natural position, as if suspended from a rope attached to the top of your head. Relax your shoulders and turn the palms of your hands to face backward.

2 Lift your heels off the floor. Let your weight move onto the balls of your feet, and pause for a moment to settle into balance in this position. Then press your hands backward, as if pushing yourself away from a wall. Your weight will now be further forward, and you will need to adjust your balance. Keep breathing naturally.

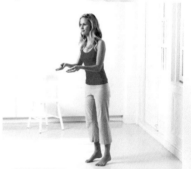

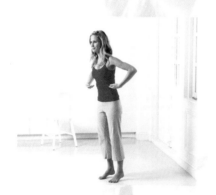

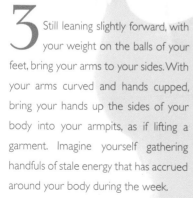

3 Still leaning slightly forward, with your weight on the balls of your feet, bring your arms to your sides. With your arms curved and hands cupped, bring your hands up the sides of your body into your armpits, as if lifting a garment. Imagine yourself gathering handfuls of stale energy that has accrued around your body during the week.

4 Bring your hands forward, palms turned upward, with your thumbs resting below the joint of your little finger. Thrust your hands forward and shake off the stale energy you've gathered up in them. Let your heels settle back onto the floor and come to rest standing with knees soft and palms now facing forward, slightly cupped.

35

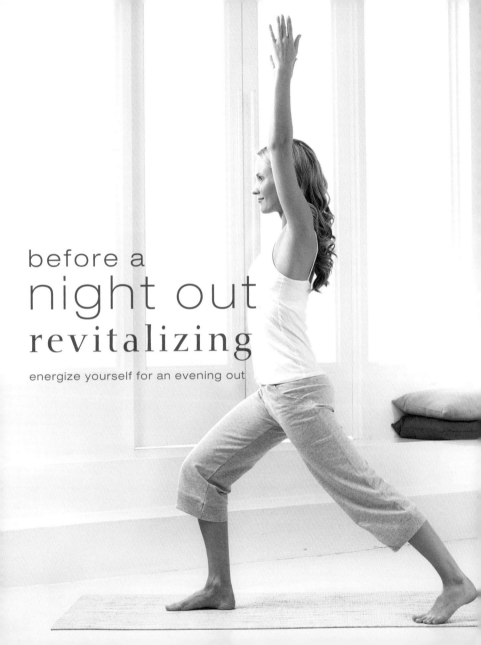

before a
night out
revitalizing

energize yourself for an evening out

1 Stand with your feet hip-width apart, arms by your sides. Check that your spine is upright, your chin slightly down, and the back of your neck long. Tuck your tailbone under slightly and keep your knees soft, not locked. Throughout this exercise, keep your pelvic muscles engaged and be careful not to arch your back.

2 *(left)* Breathe in and stride forward with your right leg, letting your left heel come off the floor. Bend your right knee, keeping your back straight. Bend your left leg if you need to. Your right knee should be no further forward than above the toes of your right foot. Raise your arms above your head, hands facing each other.

3 As you breathe out, push off strongly from your right foot and step back to your starting position. Bring your arms down at the same time. On the next in-breath, repeat the exercise, stepping forward with your left foot. If you find your back arching, take a shorter stride. Return to the start position on your outbreath.

4 Breathe in and lunge back with your right foot, keeping your right heel off the floor, bending the left knee and raising your arms above your head. As you breathe out, push off from your right foot and return to your starting position. Repeat, stepping back with your left foot. Then repeat the entire sequence six to ten times.

sunday morning
regenerating

use hand reflexology and shiatsu when space is limited

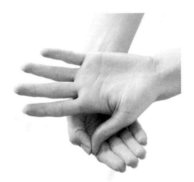

1 Like your feet, your hands have their own set of reflexology points that map your whole body. When you're feeling tired, especially from mental rather than physical work, hold your left thumb in your right hand. Press in and massage the pad of the top joint (behind the thumbnail) with your right thumb. This spot represents your brain.

2 Cradling your left hand in your right, massage all over your palm and the base of your thumb with your right thumb. Massage a point on your palm a thumb-width below your little finger. This covers the internal organs and increases energy. Rub the outside of your thumb, for the spine. Repeat steps 1 and 2 on your right hand.

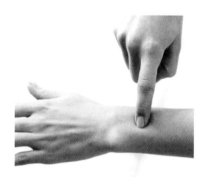

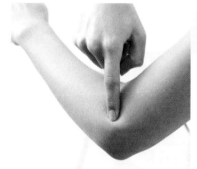

3 The ancient Chinese practice of acupressure, known as shiatsu in Japan, also makes use of energizing points that are easy to locate and work on unobtrusively. Holding your wrist, find a point three finger-widths down the back of your arm from your hand. Use your index finger to press firmly into that spot and massage it.

4 Follow an invisible line up the back of your arm and press into a spot at the outside fold of your elbow. This is easiest to find if your arm is resting, palm down, on a table in front of you. Acupressure points are often felt as a slight dip, so feel around gently to locate this, then press and massage it. This spot will give you an energy boost.

39

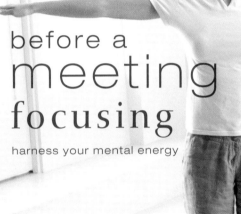

before a
meeting
focusing
harness your mental energy

1 Stand tall and look ahead of you, blinking as often as you need. Bring your breath into a slow but comfortable rhythm, by breathing in to a count of five, and out to a count of five. Focus on your breath, and the feeling as it enters and leaves your body. Feel your mind letting go of scattered thoughts and coming into focus.

2 Slowly roll your shoulders backward a few times to loosen them. Raise your arms beside you to shoulder level, so that your body makes a letter T shape. Check that raising your arms hasn't lifted your shoulders too. If so, consciously drop your shoulders, keeping your arms outstretched with palms facing down.

3 *(left)* Slowly turn your head to look along your left arm as you breathe in, and at the same time, turn your left palm upward. On the outbreath, turn your head to the right. At the same time, turn your right palm up and your left palm down. So as you breathe out, you look down the length of your right arm, palm facing upward.

4 Continue with this rhythm, breathing in as you look left and out as you look right. Turn your arms with each breath, both moving at the same time, so that the arm you are looking along always has its palm facing up. Don't let your breathing become unnaturally deep. Do this for a few minutes to help your mind focus.

41

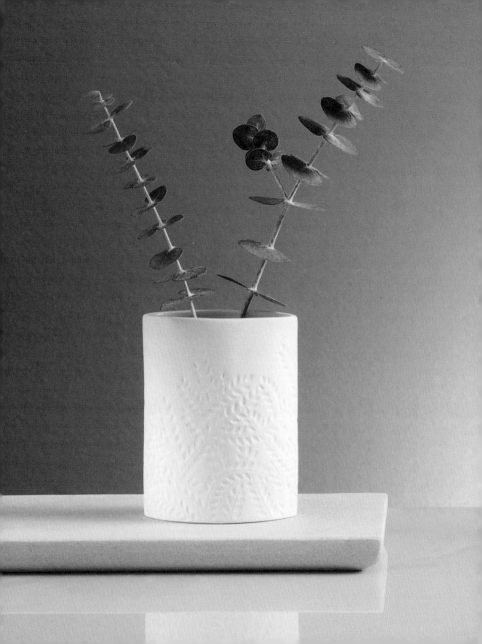

anywhere

You don't need lots of space or any special equipment to practise these simple, "anywhere" energy-boosting routines. You don't even need to leave your sofa, your car, your bathroom or your desk. Use the exercises in this chapter to pick yourself up wherever you are – so that you are always ready for action, wherever you go.

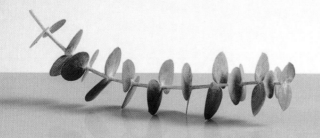

1

Lie on the floor. You may need to use a yoga mat or a towel if your floor very hard. Lie on your back with your knees bent. Adjust your position as needed to lengthen your spine. First, lift your head and try to put it back down it a little further away from your tailbone. Then raise your hips and put them down further away from your head.

2

Let your head roll from one side to the other, then come to rest in a central position, so that if you were to lift your head you would look straight down between your feet. Bring your knees up, wrap them in your arms and hug them in toward your chest.

3

Rock your hips a small distance from one side to the other. Roll them in a circular movement, increasing the roll as much as is comfortable. Gradually let your whole spine join in. Still hugging your knees, rock your whole body from side to side.

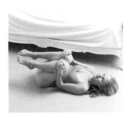

4

(right) Place your arms flat on the floor next to your sides. Lift your head and tuck in your chin. Rock forward, then let yourself roll back so that your hips come off the floor. Increase the movement until you're rolling back onto your shoulders each time, with your knees above your head. Keep your head central and your chin tucked in.

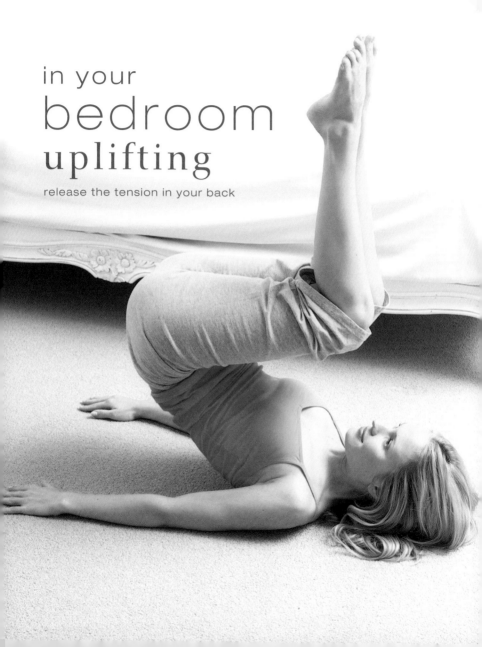

in your
bedroom
uplifting
release the tension in your back

on your sofa
replenishing

take a break and work on your pressure points

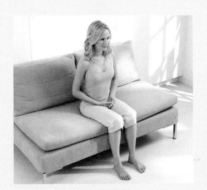 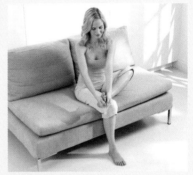

1 If dashing around has left you feeling dizzy with exhaustion, sit down and take a well earned break. Start by sitting with your feet flat on the ground for a couple of minutes. Rest your hands in your lap. Fix your eyes on something immobile in the middle distance, and focus squarely on that. Blink as often as you need.

2 After three or four breaths, take off your shoes, then rub your palms together to generate warmth. Cup your left foot in both hands. Place your right palm so that it covers part of the sole and ball of your foot, as the spot where they meet holds an important energizing acupressure point. Feel the warmth flowing into the area.

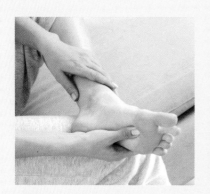

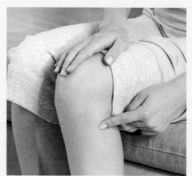

3 Find the point where your sole meets the ball of your foot, right in the centre where there is a natural dip. This is an important acupressure point, and is believed to contain a lot of energy. Working on this pressure point is said to heal dizziness. Massage it in small circles using the pad of your thumb. Repeat on the other foot.

4 If you need a burst of energy, find the spot four finger-widths down from the bottom of your kneecap, on the side of each leg. You should be able to feel a dip between the shinbone and the muscle beside it. Use your index finger to press into this point, which is said to give enough energy to walk an extra three miles.

47

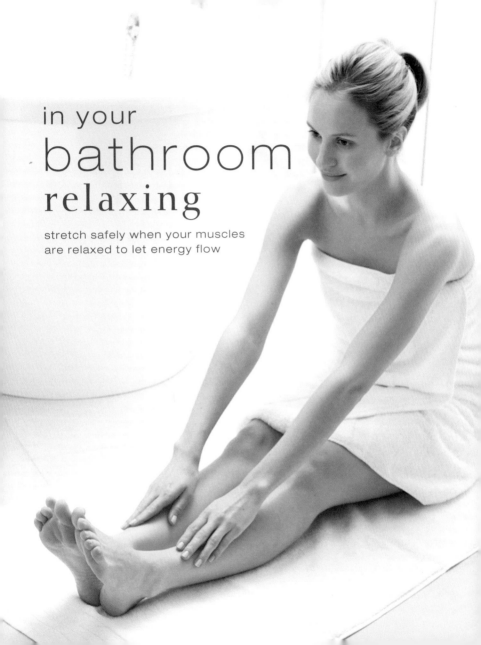

in your
bathroom
relaxing

stretch safely when your muscles
are relaxed to let energy flow

1 Light a candle and run a warm bath. Make sure that the bathroom itself is warm too, as cold air can make muscles contract again. Enjoy a relaxing bath, letting the warm water ease the day's tension out of your muscles. Then towel yourself dry and stretch while your muscles are still warm and supple.

2 Sit upright, with your legs stretched out in front of you, toes pointing up, heels pressing down. Your arms should be by your side and your back straight. Push down with your hands beside you. Inhale and lengthen upward. Keeping your torso lifted, exhale and start to lean forward, leading with your chest.

3 *(left)* Lean forward slowly, without straining your lower back. You should feel the stretch in the back of your legs only. Each time you inhale, try to lift and lengthen the front of your body. As you exhale, sink further down into the stretch. Finally, let your shoulders and head come forward and reach for your feet.

4 Hold the stretch for a few moments. Then lift your chest and come up slowly without letting your back sag. Bring your arms back to your sides and push down to help bring your torso up without slumping. Then lie on your back and bring your knees in to your chest, tuck in your chin and hug your knees.

49

in your kitchen
activating

revive your energy through chi gung

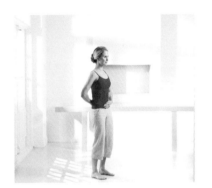

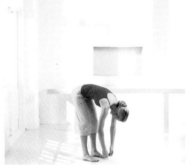

1 Stand with your feet set about hip-width apart. Your knees should be soft – not bent, but ensure that they are not rigidly locked, to avoid putting undue strain on your lower back. Arch your back, then reverse the arch by tucking your tailbone under as far as it will go. Finally come to a neutral position between the two.

2 Fold forward from your hips, letting your arms dangle down in front of you. Keep your legs strong and straight, with your feet firmly rooted. If this makes you feel dizzy, only bring your hands down as far as the kitchen worktop, standing far enough away to allow room to make your arms and back form a straight line.

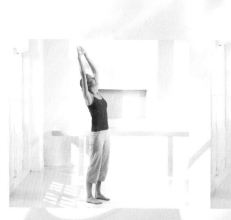

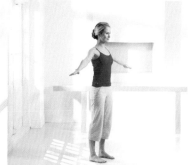

3 On an in-breath, come up slowly, raising your arms in front of you. Continue the move until you are leaning slightly backward. Don't let your lower back slump, compressing your spinal discs. Instead, keep the energy and upward movement in your spine. Bend your elbows outward and join your hands at the thumbs and index fingers.

4 After a few breaths, slowly return to the upright position with your arms above your head as you breathe in. On the next out-breath, slowly bring your arms down beside you to chest level. Pause to check that your shoulders are relaxed, not hunched up. Adjust your position if necessary. Then bring your arms down to your sides.

51

1 Turn away from your computer screen, so that it can't distract you while you're taking a much needed break. Sit with your feet flat on the floor, or stand with your back straight. Lift your shoulders and drop them a couple of times to release built-up tension: shoulders often become hunched while you're working at a screen.

2 Interlace your fingers and stretch your arms out in front of you. Adjust your position if your shoulders have crept upward again. Feel the stretch across your back, and hold this position for a few breaths. Turn your hands so your knuckles are facing you, and stretch forward again.

3 With arms still outstretched, swing your interlaced hands above your head, palms upward. Relax your elbows and drop your shoulders. Straighten your arms and stretch strongly toward the ceiling. Still facing forward and stretching upward, bend to the right and to the left.

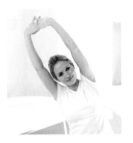

4 (right) Bring your arms down in front of you, again to shoulder-height. Keeping your hips facing forward, turn from the waist and take your outstretched arms round to your left and then to your right. Hold each stretch for a few breaths. Repeat this exercise every hour or so, whenever you are working at a desk.

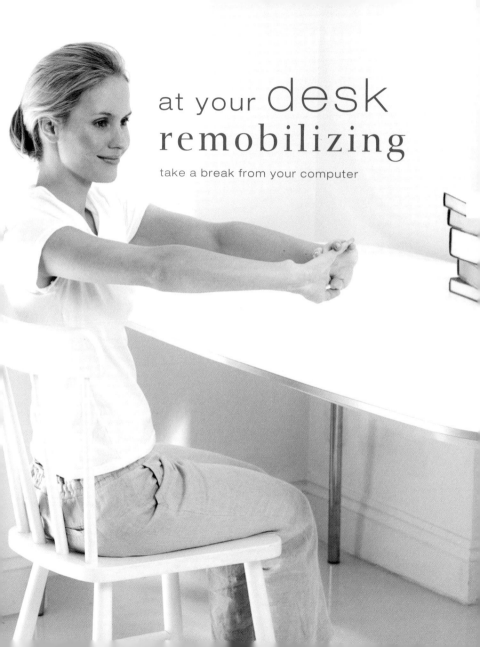

at your desk
remobilizing

take a break from your computer

in a hotel recuperating

recover quickly after travelling

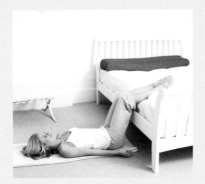 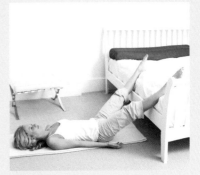

1 Put your luggage out of the way and take off your shoes. Lie down with your back on the floor and at right angles to the bed. Lie on a towel if the floor is very hard. Bend your knees, raise your feet and rest them on the bed. Let your arms relax by your sides, with your palms turned up. Feel your spine slowly relaxing and sinking into the floor.

2 After a few minutes, begin to extend your legs out sideways. Move each foot a short distance at a time to avoid a sudden groin strain. Keep extending your legs until they are in the widest V shape that doesn't hurt the insides of your thighs. Rest your feet firmly on the bed, and relax into this stretch for a few breaths.

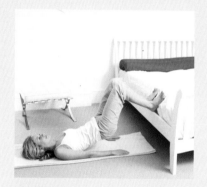 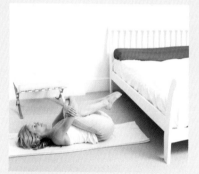

3 Come out of this leg stretch carefully. Moving your feet slowly, bring them back to hip-width apart on the bed. Turn your hands palm down on the floor. Pressing your feet against the bed, raise your lower back slightly off the floor. If the bed begins to move, do this with your feet flat on the floor instead. Hold this stretch for two breaths.

4 Curl your spine onto the floor again, trying to put each vertebra down gradually, one by one. Bring your knees in to your chest, keep your head central and hug your knees to your body. Repeat steps 3 and 4 twice, each time aiming for a small and controlled arch in the spine when you raise it, and a gentle return to the floor.

55

1 Stand up, rise onto your toes and then sit down again. March on the spot if you have room. Sitting still for a long time can make you feel lethargic, so keep your muscles working regularly. Take the opportunity to walk around the plane whenever possible.

2 Sit with your feet flat on the floor, back straight. Raise and lower your heels, keeping the balls of your feet on the floor. Tighten your calf muscle as your heel comes up. Raise one after the other, then both together. Then raise your heels higher, so you come onto your toes.

3 Sitting with your left knee raised, point your toes down to the floor and then flex your foot so that your toes point upward. Extend the movement to the whole of your lower leg, bringing it forward when you point your toes and then back again when you flex your foot.

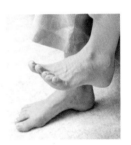

Next rotate your ankle in both directions, swivelling your ankle to the greatest degree possible. Repeat this step with your right leg and foot.

4 *(right)* Cradling your left foot in your right hand, imagine a line running from the centre of your big toe pad to the lower corner of the next toe. Press firmly halfway along this line. According to reflexology, working on this spot reduces travel exhaustion. Repeat on your right foot.

on a plane
clearing

combat travel exhaustion
and encourage blood flow

1 To combat lethargy when driving, take the chance to massage your ears when you're in a traffic jam or when waiting at traffic lights. According to Chinese medicine, the whole body is represented by points on the ear, so ear massage provides all-over energy. Start by folding your ear over to cover the opening.

2 *(right)* Find the point where your ear joins your scalp at the top, and pinch it gently between your index finger and your thumb. Lift your fingers off and then repeat this movement just below. Work your way around the edge of your ear from top to bottom, pinching and releasing. Do it again, increasing the pressure.

3 Repeat this gentle pinching movement over your whole ear, as far as you can reach. It should feel stimulating but not painful. Massage your earlobes. Put your thumbs carefully into the whorls of your ears and massage the whole area. Put your index finger in your ear and make small circles. Repeat on your other ear.

4 Hold your earlobes firmly and pull forward, backward and then downward. Work your way round the edge of your ear, pulling backward. Hold the top of your ears and pull upward. Repeat steps 1 to 4 two or three times. However, if you find that you are beginning to feel really sleepy, pull over and take a break.

58

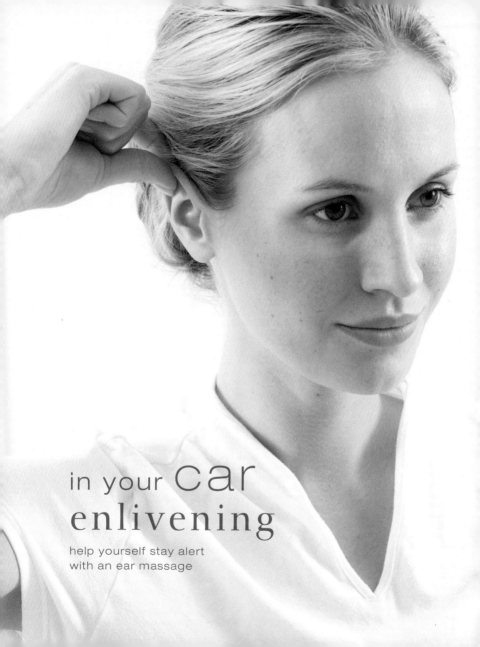

in your car
enlivening

help yourself stay alert
with an ear massage

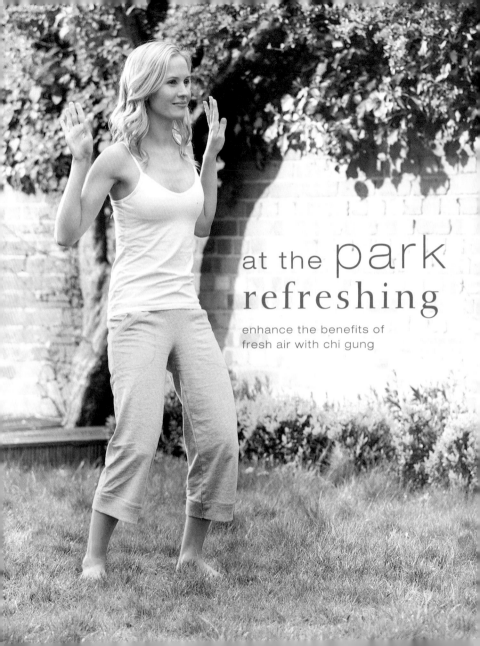

at the park
refreshing

enhance the benefits of
fresh air with chi gung

1 Stand with your knees soft, tailbone tucked under, and feet hip-width apart. Keeping your shoulders relaxed, raise your arms in front of you, palms facing down, as you breathe in. When they reach shoulder level, bend your knees slightly. Breathing out, bring your arms toward your body, with elbows down and wrists up.

2 As you breathe in, straighten your legs. At the same time, stretch your arms out in front of you again. This time raise your hands, palms facing away from you, as if you were gently pushing something away. Breathe out and lower your arms back down to your sides. Repeat steps 1 and 2 several times.

3 *(left)* With arms hanging loosely, turn your palms inward. This time raise them out beside you to make a T shape. As you breathe in, slowly raise them to shoulder-level. Keep your shoulders low and relaxed. On the outbreath, bend your knees slightly and drop your elbows, bringing your hands in toward your shoulders.

4 Breathe in as you straighten your arms and legs. Stand tall and push outward to the sides, fingers pointing up. Then bend your knees and bring your arms in on an outbreath. Continue with this wave-like movement for several more breaths, visualizing an increase of positive energy moving around your body.

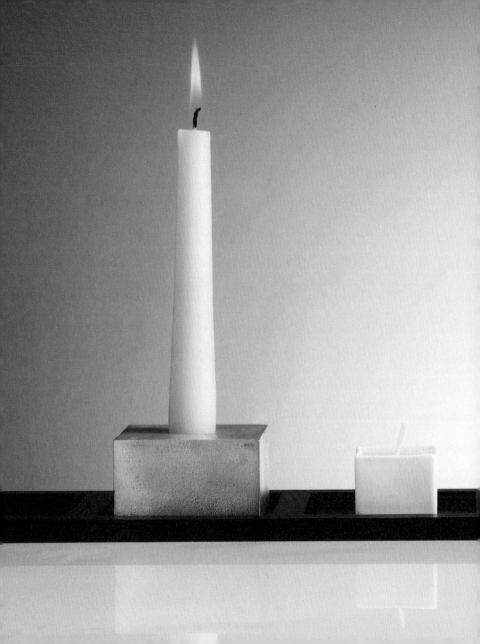

body energizers

Your body produces energy and uses energy, but it can trap energy, too – whether that's deep within your muscles or at specific points on your subtle body. All the techniques in this chapter, from massage and breath control to voice exercises and aerobics, aim to release energy from specific parts of your body, enabling it to flow freely again.

1 Raise your arms and hold your head – put the heels of your hands on your hairline, fingers stretching back across your scalp. Without lifting your hands, move them in large circles. Press hard enough to move your scalp over your skull, but without pulling your hair.

2 Starting from your hairline, press your fingers against your scalp and make small circles. Again, aim to move skin over bone rather than stretching your hair. Lift your fingers and repeat the movement all over your head. If your scalp is very tense, it may feel uncomfortable at first.

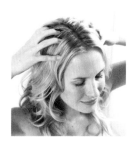

3 *(right)* Put your hands on the back of your head, fingers pointing upward. Gently press in to move your scalp upward over your skull. Explore with your thumbs to locate the ridge at the bottom of your skull, roughly level with your ears. When you have found it, massage gently all the way along it using the pads of your thumbs.

4 Run your fingers lightly across your scalp as if dividing your hair into sections. If your nails aren't too long, crook your fingers slightly so that you are working with the tips of your fingers. Include some very slight nail pressure. Run your fingers through the full length of your hair, lifting it and letting it fall. Repeat all over your scalp.

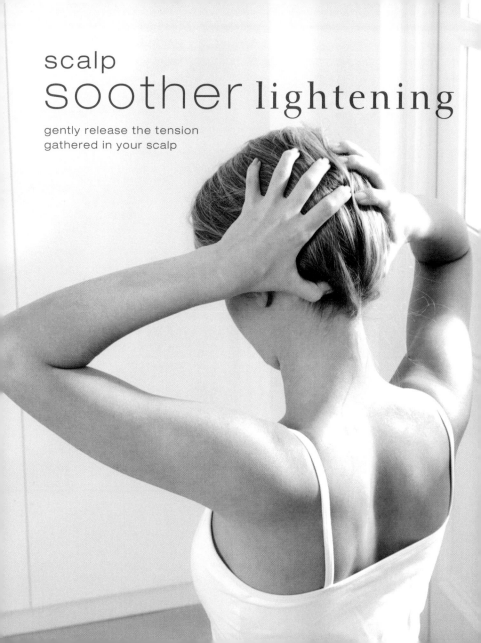

scalp
soother lightening

gently release the tension
gathered in your scalp

face lifter
toning

wake up your skin with an ayurvedic marma-point massage

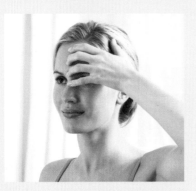 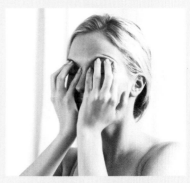

1 Press your ring finger into the point between your eyebrows, the middle finger just above it and the index finger close to the hairline. Lift your fingers and press again, one finger-width to the side. Using both hands, continue this movement out across your forehead and temples, pressing slowly in against the bone, not up or down.

2 Feel for the upper edge of your eye sockets, and carefully press the bone with all eight fingertips. Place your fingers just above your eye sockets and press again, this time pushing upward so your forehead furrows. Place the flat of your middle finger below the centre of your eyes on the edge of your eye socket. Apply light pressure.

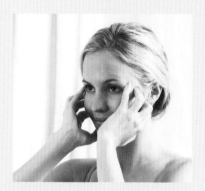 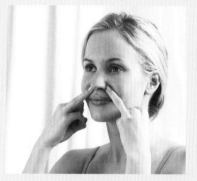

3 Find a point directly below the cheekbone, still in line with the centre of your eyes. Press upward into the bottom of your cheekbone. Put the flat of each little finger on the socket beside the outer edge of each eye, and spread the other fingers out along a diagonal line to the bottom of your ear lobe. Press with all eight fingers.

4 Find a point at the outer edge of each nostril, and press firmly diagonally inward with your ring fingers. Next, bunch all eight fingers close together so that you can press along the space between your top lip and your nose. Do the same below your lower lip. Finally, press the tip of one thumb into the centre of your chin.

FACE LIFTER

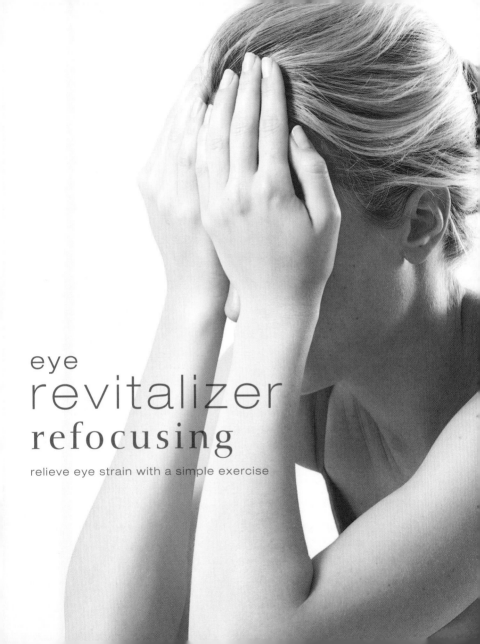

eye
revitalizer
refocusing
relieve eye strain with a simple exercise

1 If your eyes start to feel dry or scratchy, take a break. Fill your hands with cool water and splash it over your face and eyes. Repeat this several times. Make sure you're drinking enough water, too, as dehydration can affect not only your eyes, but also your energy levels. Blink frequently to spread soothing tears across your eyeballs.

2 Awaken your eye muscles by using them to their full capacity. Instead of constantly focusing at the same distance, let your eyes settle on something at the other side of the room. Then look at something nearby. Finally, look out of the window and give your eyes a few moments to focus on a distant object.

3 Turn your head to the left, and focus on whatever forms the horizon where you are – probably a wall. Very slowly turn your head all the way to the right. Your eyes should not move, just allow them to be carried along by the movement of your head. Let your focus sweep along without making any effort.

4 Rub your hands together to warm them. Then lift your hands up to your face and rest your face in your hands. Cup your hands around your eyes so that all light is excluded. Open your eyes and let them rest in the warm, dark space. Visualize a place where you feel happy, and relax for a few minutes.

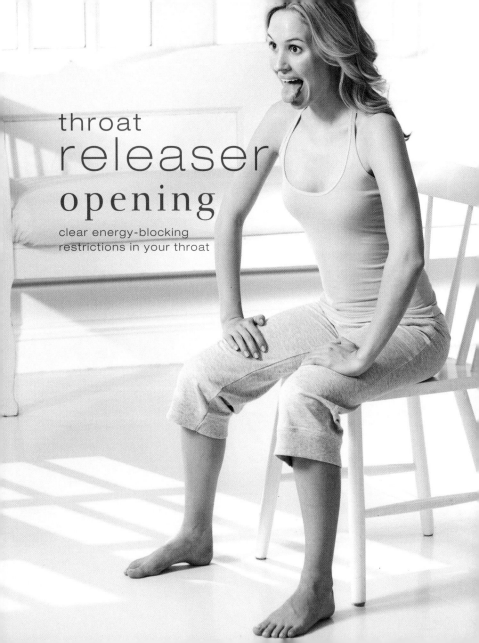

throat
releaser
opening

clear energy-blocking
restrictions in your throat

1 Tension in the throat can be the cause of tight muscles around the jaw or even a weak voice. It also creates a bottleneck for energy. Unblock your energy by doing voice exercises. Start by breathing into your abdomen: put your hand there and feel air push it out as you breathe in. It may feel unnatural at first.

2 Start humming a simple tune. Explore the feeling in your throat and the back of your mouth. Notice the reverberation of different notes. Now open your mouth and make a quiet "hah" sound. Let the sound last for your entire out-breath. Be careful not to breathe in too deeply; the out-breath can last longer.

3 Now take a deep breath and let it out with a long sigh. Continue with a few loud, exaggerated sighs. Make each one louder and longer than the one before. Then, do some long fake yawns. Soon they will be real yawns, easing tension out of your jaw. Be careful at this point not to breathe so deeply that you become dizzy.

4 *(left)* Sit on a chair and lean slightly forward, legs apart and hands on thighs, fingers pointing inward. Breathe out with a loud "hah" sound, opening your mouth and eyes wide. Push your tongue right out. Splay out your fingers and look fierce. Relax as you breathe in. Repeat three times, making the "hah" louder each time.

1 Stand with your feet hip-width apart, knees slightly bent. Keep your back straight without arching your waist. Lift and drop your shoulders to relax them. As you breathe in, bring both hands up in front of your chest, elbows out to the side, palms facing away from you.

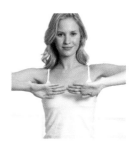

2 *(right)* As you breathe out, push your left hand out in front of you. Keep your arm at shoulder height. When your arm is almost straight, turn the palm back toward your face. As you breathe in, bring the left palm back toward your chest. At the same time, push your right hand out in front of you, palm facing away from you.

3 Halfway through this in-breath, you should see your left palm coming toward your chest, and the back of your right hand moving away. At the end of each outward movement, turn your hand so that it faces you on the way back. Just before your palm reaches your chest, turn it to face away from you on the outward journey.

4 Breathing at a slow but natural pace, try to harmonize your movements with your breath. One arm movement out and in should coincide with one breath out and in. Keep checking your posture and make sure that your shoulders haven't become tense and raised.

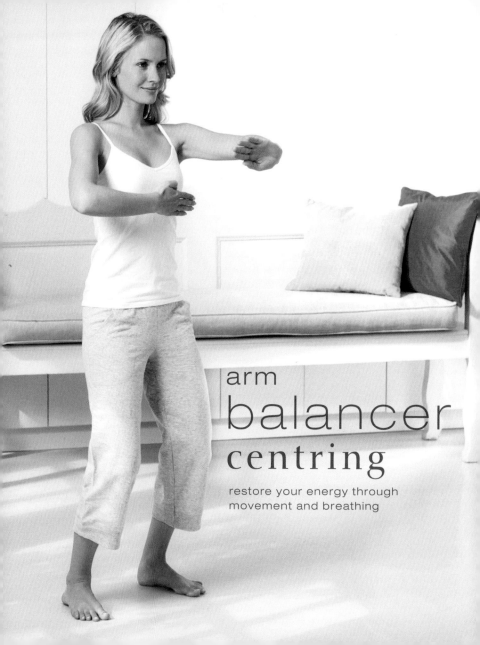

arm
balancer
centring

restore your energy through
movement and breathing

1 Sit with your back straight but not rigid, your hands relaxed on your thighs. Lift and drop your shoulders a few times to release some of the stiffness or residual tension stored in them. Close your eyes and try to lengthen your spine upward, feeling as if a little space is opening up between each of your vertebrae.

2 *(right)* When your spine feels lengthened, take a deep breath and stretch your arms out to the sides. Feel your back growing wider as it releases the muscle tension holding it tight and pinched. Wrap your arms around your chest to hug yourself. Bring your shoulders as far forward as you can without discomfort.

3 Put your hands on your hips. Slide them backward, until your thumbs are beside your spine. Press into the muscles beside the spine. These are acupressure points used for relieving exhaustion. It is thought to improve the circulation of both blood and chi to the kidneys and, indeed, the back in general.

4 Using the pads of your thumbs, massage the big muscles on either side of your spinal column in small circles. Don't put any pressure on the spine itself, but work instead on the muscles that support it. Then move your hands up, finger-width by finger-width, massaging as far up your back as you can.

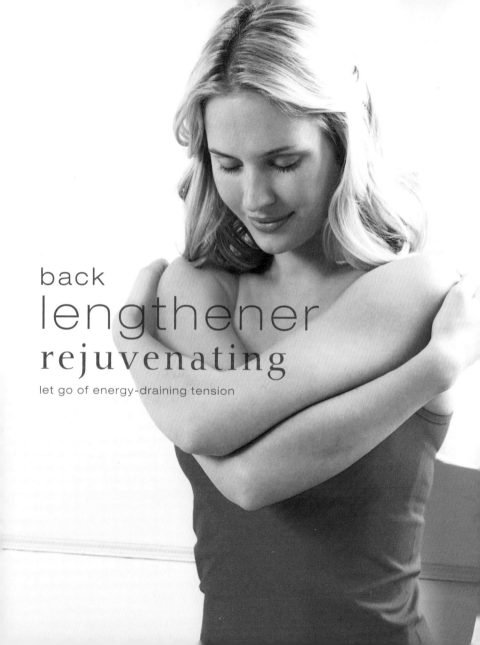

back
lengthener
rejuvenating

let go of energy-draining tension

leg invigorator
energizing

revive the circulation in your legs

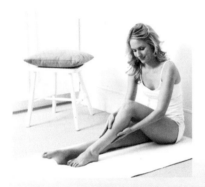

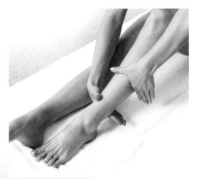

1 These massage steps can be done on top of clothes, wherever you are. But for the most luxurious effects, pour a teaspoonful of your favourite oil into your cupped hands, rub it into your palms, and slowly massage into your bare legs, avoiding any visible veins. Begin by taking a seat with your legs stretched comfortably out in front of you.

2 Make an L shape with your left thumb and index finger. Using this as your massage tool, run it up the upper surface of your left leg. Use long, firm strokes, starting at your ankle. Using your right hand in the same way, make firm strokes up the back of your leg. Next, work up the sides. Change hands and do the same on your right leg.

76

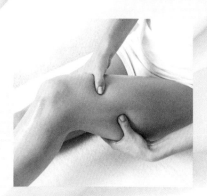

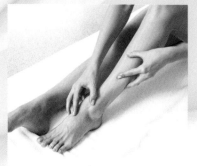

3 Using your thumbs and index fingers, grip your calf muscle just above the ankle. Squeeze and massage in circles, especially anywhere that feels tired or tight. Lift your hand and repeat two finger-widths higher up, and continue up your leg toward your groin. Use both hands to massage your thigh, working from each side.

4 Place your fingers on the front and back of your ankles, keeping your fingers loose and slightly curved. Run your hands firmly up your leg, using long strokes from your ankles to your groin. Use the soft pads of your fingers rather than the tips. Do the same up the sides of your legs. Repeat several times on both legs.

1 Rest your right ankle on your left knee. Hold your right foot in both hands, with your two thumbs on the sole. Massage the centre of the sole just below the ball of your foot – an acupressure point said to boost energy. Continue over your sole, toes, and the sides and top of your foot.

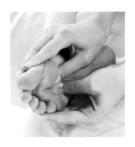

2 *(right)* With your thumbs back on your sole, gently move the sides of your foot up and down as if trying to fold it. Circle your ankle. Gently pull each toe. Interlace your toes with your fingers as far as you can go without forcing your toes uncomfortably apart. Move your hand in a circle to mobilize your toes. Repeat steps 1 and 2 on your left foot.

3 Fill two bowls with enough water to immerse your feet and ankles – one with cool water, the other with warm water. Test the temperature by dipping in the tip of your elbow. You can add a few drops of energizing essential oil, such as basil, geranium, rosemary, pine or thyme to the warm bowl. These are all said to relieve tiredness.

4 Immerse your feet for a couple of minutes in the warm footbath. Massage the water gently into your feet. Then swap to the cool bowl. Splash cold water on your ankles while your feet are soaking. Use each bowl two or three times, then dry your feet and put on warm socks.

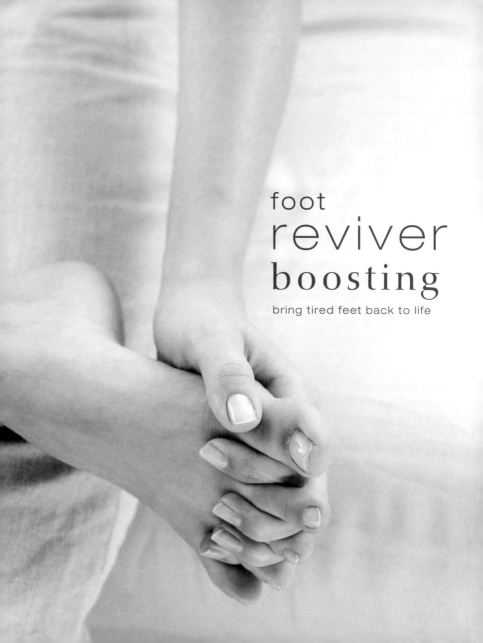

foot
reviver
boosting

bring tired feet back to life

body booster
enhancing

encourage your lymph and blood circulation

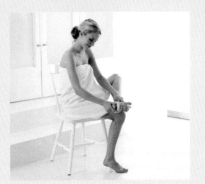
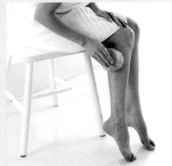

1 Start by rinsing and drying your feet. Using a firm brush made from natural bristles, brush the sole of one foot four to six times, starting from your toes and working toward your ankle. Press firmly enough not to tickle but not hard enough to hurt. Repeat the brushing movement on the sides and top of your foot, using long strokes.

2 Work your way up your leg, finishing by brushing toward the lymph glands in your groin. Repeat this process on your other foot and leg. Continue with long, firm brush strokes up your buttocks, hips and back. Brush gently in circles around your abdomen and then up over your stomach and chest into your armpits.

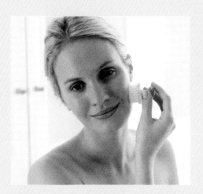

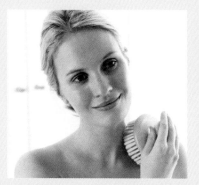

3 For your face, use a very soft-bristled brush or an exfoliating pad. Be careful not to drag your skin. Working from the centre of your face, brush outward across your forehead toward your temples. Brush down your nose, out across your cheeks toward your ears, and out along your jaw. Work toward the lymph glands in your neck.

4 Use a body brush to work down your neck, throat, upper back and upper chest toward your armpits. Make gentle semi-circular movements on your chest, working from your nipples into your armpits. Brush your hands and arms as you did your feet and legs. Steps 1 to 4 can be done every morning for a few minutes. Then shower thoroughly.

all-over blitzer motivating

give yourself a burst of energy in a sedentary day

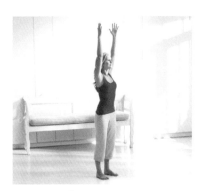

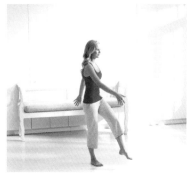

1 When you're feeling jaded after sitting down for too long, take a few minutes to re-energize. Start by standing up and stretching your arms as high as you can reach. Breathe in deeply as you do so. As you breathe out, bring your arms out to the sides and down. Repeat two or three times.

2 Raise your shoulders toward your ears and let them fall. Repeat twice to ensure your shoulders aren't holding tension. Then raise your arms and shake them. Bring them down to your sides, still shaking them. Raise one leg at a time and shake the tension out of your leg muscles.

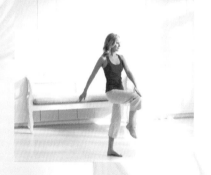

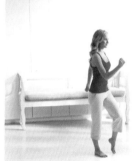

3 Start walking on the spot, kicking your foot out in front of you at each step. Then raise your right knee and tap it with your left hand. Repeat with your left knee and right hand. Continue this marching step, speeding up till you start to breathe faster. If you become too breathless to speak, slow down!

4 Bend your left knee and lift your left heel. Put your left heel down, then raise your right heel and bend your right knee. Repeat a few times, then speed up so that you're "running" on the spot without lifting your toes off the ground. Move your arms as if really running. Slow down gradually and stop.

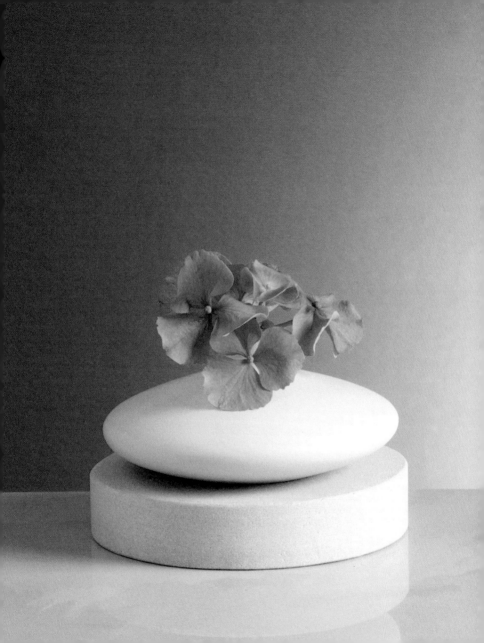

mood enhancers

Your mental processes have a powerful effect on your body. Think about how stress saps your energy, whereas happiness and excitement create an energy surge. The techniques in this chapter will help you to lift your spirits, calm your anxiety and refocus your scattered thoughts – all with the ultimate aim of making you feel positive and full of life.

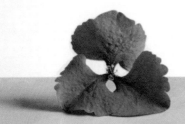

1 Put on a dance CD, or any music that has a fast, lively rhythm. Sway your upper body from side to side as the music washes away the stress of your day. Continue to sway your upper body, but now swing your arms and tap your feet too. Concentrate on the rhythm of the music.

2 (right) Continue with some hip-swinging moves. Step to the right then bring your left foot next to your right foot. Repeat this move for three more sideways steps. On the fourth step, don't put your left foot down, just tap your toes. Then step to the left, close up with the right and repeat till you're back where you started. Repeat three times in each direction.

3 On the next step to the right, take a quarter turn. Complete the full clockwise turn in four small steps. Repeat the basic routine as in step 2, then make another full turn in four small steps. Keep your elbows near your sides, hands raised to waist level, and move your arms to the beat.

4 Next step back on your right foot, then rock forward on your left. Bring your right foot back beside the left, and tap your left foot. Step forward with your left foot, rock back onto your right, bring your left foot beside the right, and tap your right foot. Repeat all the moves eight times.

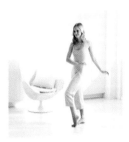

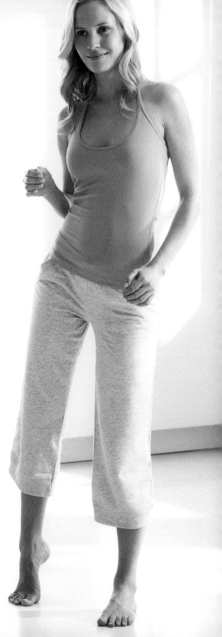

mood lifter
cheering

revive low spirits fast with
energizing dancing

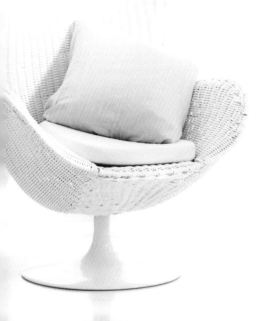

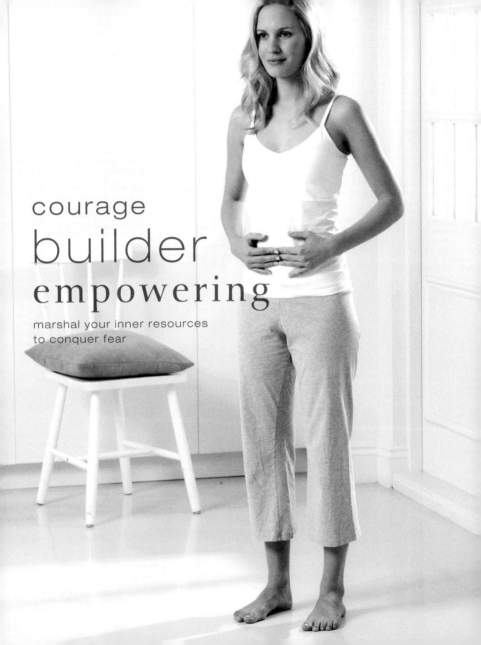

courage
builder
empowering

marshal your inner resources
to conquer fear

1 Stand with your feet slightly apart so that you have a stable base. Lift your toes, one foot at a time, spread them out and plant your feet more firmly on the ground. Feel them well grounded. Close your eyes and visualize roots growing down from your feet, tapping the strength and solidity of the earth.

2 Use the whole of your lungs to breathe. Don't take unnaturally deep breaths, but just allow the air to flow right down into the depths of your lungs. Put your right hand on your chest and your left hand on your abdomen; you should be able to feel your abdomen moving out as you take each breath in.

3 Breathe in slowly to the count of four. Breathe out slowly to the same count. Establishing this steady regular pattern, visualize strength and courage flooding into your body as the air fills your lungs. As you breathe out, visualize negativity and fear leaving your body.

4 *(left)* Put both of your hands on your abdomen. Find the point three finger-widths below your navel – this is your body's centre. Focus your mind on this spot, as you steadily breathe the earth's strength into your centre. Finally, straighten your back, lift your head and smile.

COURAGE BUILDER

mental refresher
inspiring

sharpen your senses with chi gung

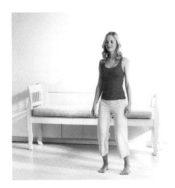

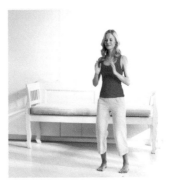

1 Stand with your feet hip-width apart, feeling relaxed but grounded. Your knees should be very slightly bent, your arms loose and your back upright in its natural curve. Bend your elbows until your forearms are vertical, hands in front of your chest. Your palms should be facing each other.

2 Visualize a ball of golden energy between your hands. Imagine that you can feel the ball in your hands. Feel the warmth on your palms. Test the edge of this ball by moving your palms slowly toward and away from each other, a couple of centimetres (one inch) at a time, as if squeezing a beach ball.

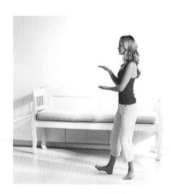

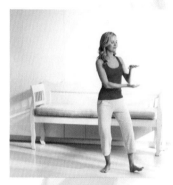

3 Lift your right toes and slowly rotate to the right on your heel. Turn your whole body, bending your left knee to prevent strain. As you turn, rotate the "ball". When you put your toes back on the floor, your right hand should be at chest level, palm down, your left hand at waist level, palm up.

4 Lift your right toes and slowly rotate left back to the central position, rotating the ball at the same time. Repeat the movement to your left, turning the ball with your left hand above and your right hand below. Concentrate on channelling the feeling of energy between your palms.

91

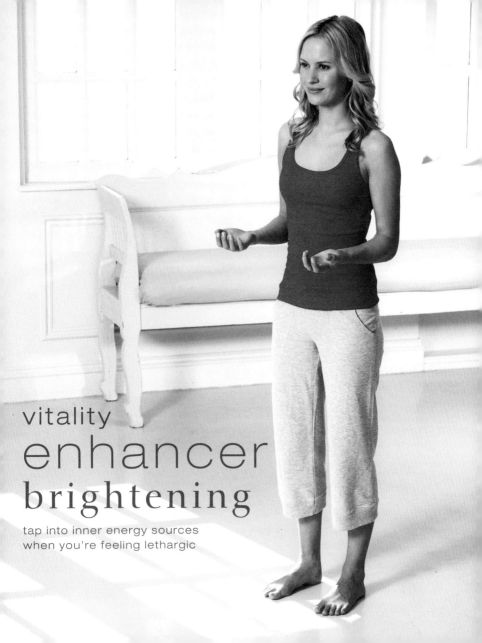

vitality
enhancer
brightening

tap into inner energy sources
when you're feeling lethargic

1 Lift and drop your shoulders to relax your muscles. With your arms loose by your sides, shake your hands as if turning a tap rapidly on and off. Lift your hands up to your shoulders and drop them several times, as if shaking off water. Lift your shoulders and hands and let your hands fall to shake out any last tension.

2 *(left)* Turn the palms of your hands upward. Make each hand into a fist, and then stretch your fingers and thumbs outward as far as possible. Feel the energy circulating through your hands. Then relax them and let your fingers curve slightly as if holding a large ball in each hand. They should feel energetic but not rigid.

3 Bring your fingers in toward your chest. Keeping your wrists loose throughout, swing your hands forward to tap your chest with all your fingers. Continue in a light drumming motion. Tapping the breastbone just below the collar bones is said to increase vitality.

4 Spread out to tap across your chest in a light, rhythmic pattern. This lively movement can be continued all over your body, including your scalp and face. Tap gently over your face, but work more forcefully across your shoulders and back, taking care to avoid the vertebrae.

1
Sit on a chair that's the right height for you to put your feet flat on the floor, slightly apart. Round your shoulders and then reverse the position by arching your back. Move from one position to the other and come into a central position, with your back naturally upright.

2
Close your eyes and raise your hands in front of your chest as if you were holding a ball. Imagine you have a ball of energy between your hands. Press inwards as if squeezing it, feeling some resistance between your hands. Your fingers should be relaxed but not floppy.

3
Keeping that feeling of energy in your hands, put one palm on the small of your back – a key acupressure point. Press firmly, feeling the warmth replenishing your energy. With finger and thumb, massage small circles into the muscles beside your spine. This will help your chi to flow freely.

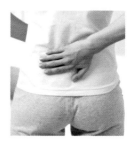

4
(right) Rub your palms together to rekindle the warmth. Then place them one above the other on your abdomen, directly below your navel. They will be covering two other acupressure points: one a couple of finger-widths up from your pubic bone and the other – your body's centre – about three finger-widths below your navel. Working on these points opens your body's energy gates and restores your innate strength.

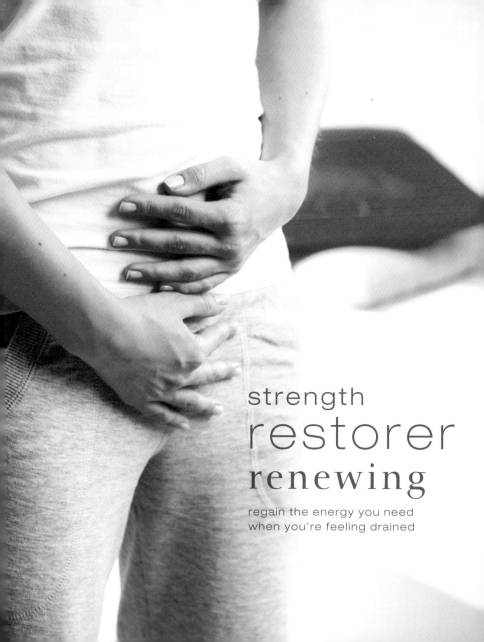

strength
restorer
renewing

regain the energy you need
when you're feeling drained

energy giver
humouring

shake off feelings of irritation

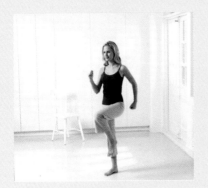 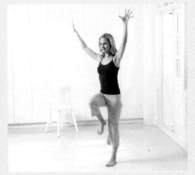

1 Whenever you become annoyed by something you can't change, work off your feelings by marching on the spot as if walking away from the problem. Swing your arms with elbows bent and fists pumping. March briskly, raising your knees and bringing your heels down at each step.

2 Continue to march on the spot. Roll your shoulders in circles to relieve any tension stored in them. Then fling your arms up toward the sky in time with your footsteps. Splay your fingers out as they reach the top of the movement. Bring them down to shoulder-level and fling them up again.

96

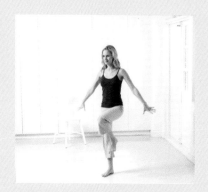 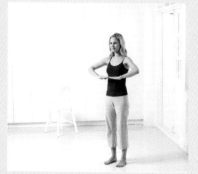

3 Keep marching on the spot. As your arms come down to shoulder-level, continue the movement until your fingers are pointing down at the floor. Open your fingers again and shake them as if you were throwing something away. Visualize throwing your irritation out of your hands.

4 Gradually slow down and come to a halt, hands by your sides. Take a few slow breaths, bringing the air down to the bottom of your lungs. As you breathe in, slowly raise your hands in front of you, palms facing down and elbows out to the sides. Bring them down slowly as you breathe out.

97

1 Kneel on all fours, with your hands directly below your shoulders and your knees below your hips. Let your waist sink slightly toward the floor while you look upward, without letting your head tip back. Then raise your back and round your shoulders, letting your head drop forward.

2 Come to a central position, keeping your spine long and straight. Your neck should continue this natural line, so you'll be looking at the floor. The next time you breathe out, engage your abdominal muscles to help you to keep your balance and prevent any strain on your spine.

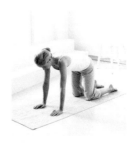

3 (*right*) Breathe in. On the next out-breath raise your left arm and stretch it out in front of you, parallel to the floor. Turn your head slightly to look at your raised arm. At the same time, raise your right leg and stretch it out as straight as possible behind you. Keep your abdominal muscles engaged to help you to hold this position without wobbling.

4 Breathe in and return to the central position. Breathe out and raise your right arm and left leg, turning to look at your right arm. Don't stretch so far that you compromise your posture or balance; the main aim is to create a steady rhythm. Continue alternating arms and legs in a fluid motion, co-ordinated with your breath.

mental
focuser
co-ordinating

practise this cross-crawl to balance mind and body

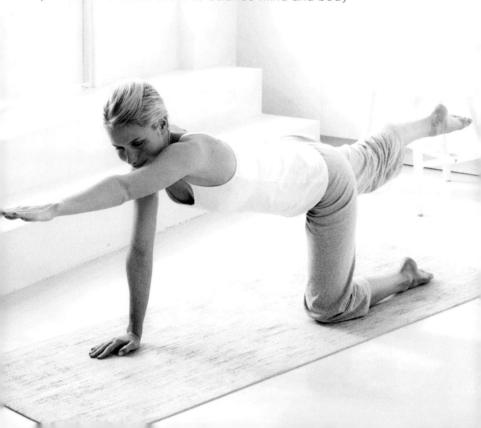

anxiety settler soothing

centre yourself fast and effectively when you're worried

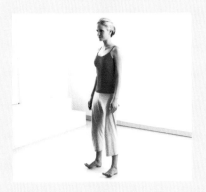 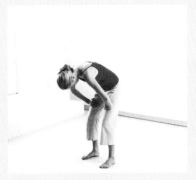

1 This exercise involves holding your breath, so don't do it if you have high blood pressure. Stand with your feet hip-width apart. Rock backward and forward on your feet and come to a central position. Feel your weight safely grounded through your hips, thighs, calves, ankles and feet.

2 Bend your knees and lean forward. Support your weight with your hands on your thighs. Aim to round your lower back and curve your spine into a gentle bow-shape. Unlike many exercises, this doesn't require a straight back. So make sure you're not leaning forward with your spine straight.

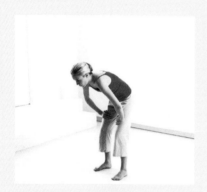

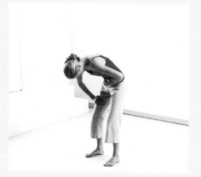

3 Take a few deep breaths and blow out to exhale the last one fully. Then hold your breath and pull your stomach in. Imagine bringing your navel up toward your spine. Focus on your body's centre, three finger-widths below your navel. Look up and pull in all your core muscles below your navel.

4 Let your muscles relax before you breathe back in again. Then exhale and pull in your muscles again. Place your hand on your stomach, over your body's centre, three finger-widths below the navel. Repeat two or three times, focusing on centring yourself with your inner resources.

101

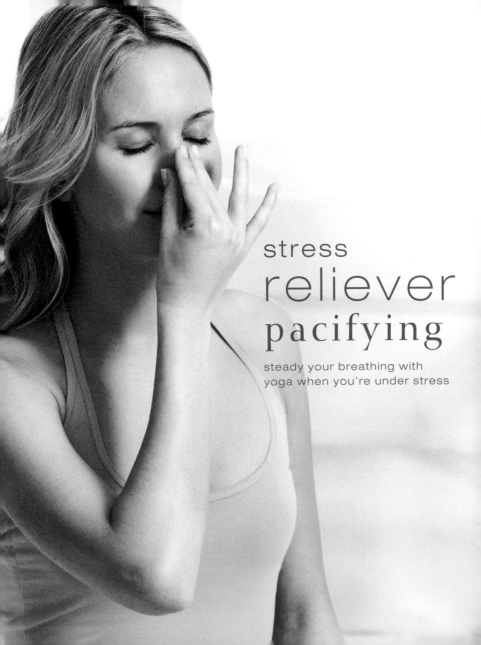

stress
reliever
pacifying

steady your breathing with
yoga when you're under stress

1 Sit comfortably with your back supported and your feet flat on the floor. Let your left hand rest in your lap (or your right, if you're left-handed). Take a few moments to rest if you've been in a hurry or coping with a stressful situation. Let your breathing slow down to a normal, steady pace.

2 Close your eyes. Place the index and second fingers of your right hand on top of your nose, pointing toward your forehead. Practise alternately covering your right nostril with your thumb and your left nostril with your ring finger, until the movement becomes easy.

3 *(left)* Close your right nostril with your thumb and breathe out steadily through the left nostril to the count of four. Inhale through the left nostril to the count of four. Keep this rhythm going throughout the entire exercise. It's an unhurried pace, but it should not feel unnaturally slow.

4 Uncover your right nostril and close your left nostril with your ring finger. Breathe out to the count of four, then inhale to the count of four, and so on. One nostril may well feel clearer than the other, which is normal. But if it seems really blocked, don't try to force it.

103

1 Sit in a quiet place where you won't be disturbed. Take a moment to relax. Put the webbing between thumb and forefinger of your left hand against the same area on the right. Then clasp your hands so your right index finger stretches down toward the wrist of your left hand.

2 Find the point your index finger reaches on the bone below the side of your thumb. You should feel a slight natural dip. Press your fingertip into this spot and keep up the pressure for several seconds. According to Chinese medicine, this shiatsu point can help to release emotion.

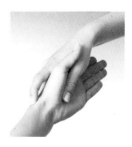

3 *(right)* To work a different shiatsu point, find a spot on the fleshy pad at the base of your left thumb, just two finger-widths up from the wrist. Using your right thumb, press in firmly against the bone, and then massage around the area, making small circles with your thumb.

4 Repeat steps 1 to 3 on your other hand. According to Chinese and Japanese medicine, these two points are good places for releasing both physical and emotional stagnation. Working on them allows blocked energy to move and frees emotions.

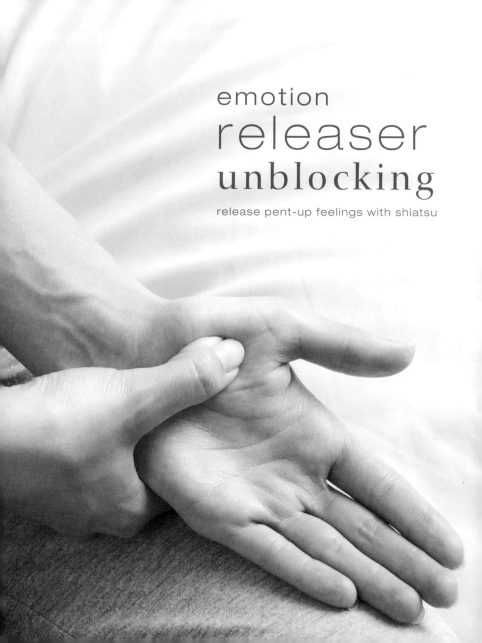

emotion
releaser
unblocking

release pent-up feelings with shiatsu

tension unwinder
loosening

stretch out to liberate blocked energy

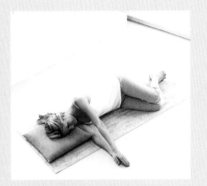 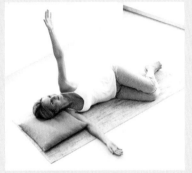

1 Lie on your right side with your knees bent, feet in line with your spine and a pillow under your head to keep your spine in alignment. Bring your hands together on the floor in front of you. To keep your pelvis square to the floor, try to bring your left hip away from your ribs and closer to your feet.

2 Keeping your hips still, raise your left hand high. Take it as far left as possible, letting your shoulders and upper body follow its movement. Don't force your left shoulder onto the floor; just let your chest open without straining your spine. Return to the starting position and repeat twice.

106

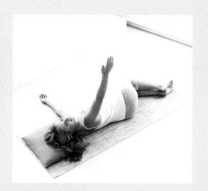 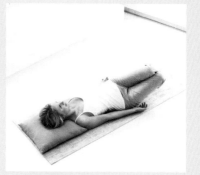

3 Roll onto your left side. Adjust your position carefully, lining up your spine with your feet and trying to push your upper hip toward your feet. Engage your abdominal muscles and repeat the exercise on the left side. Remember, the aim is to keep the hips still while moving the upper body.

4 Roll onto your back with knees bent, feet on the floor and arms by your sides. Swing your knees slowly toward the right side, then the left. Again, don't force them down to the floor. This time, keep your shoulders flat on the floor to create openness in your lower back. Repeat twice on each side.

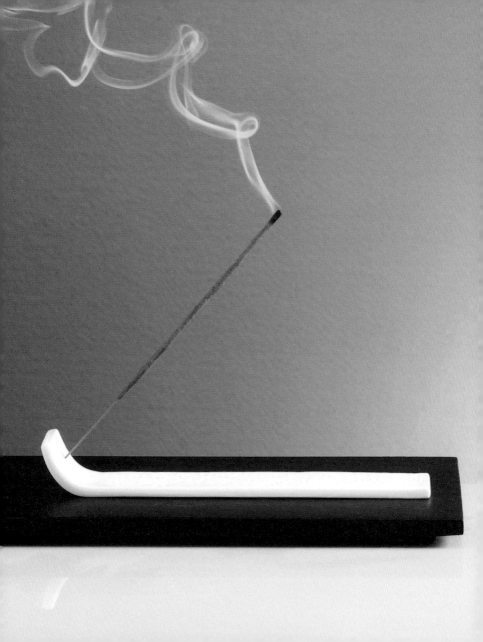

practising together

Whether it's to enhance an energizing stretch or to draw on the positive energy of your partner or friend, two often work better than one. The exercises in this chapter will help you both to make the most of all the energizing techniques in this book, and to tune into each other's energy to increase and affirm your special bond.

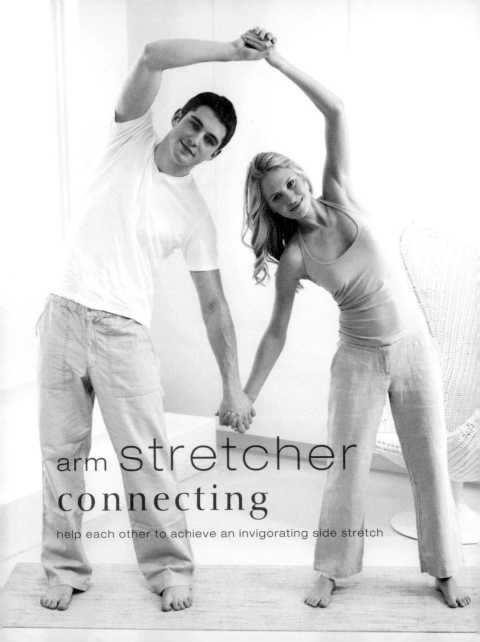

arm stretcher
connecting

help each other to achieve an invigorating side stretch

1 During this exercise, both partners do the same thing at the same time. Stand side by side, about an arm's-length apart, facing the same way. Plant your feet firmly on the ground, shoulder-width apart. Check your posture to ensure that your back is neither slumped nor arched. Lift your shoulders and let them relax.

2 Reach out with your inside hand and join hands with your partner. Raise your outside arm, palm facing toward your partner, and feel the energy coursing through your spine, arm and fingertips. Start to move your arm outward, and let the rest of your body follow it, so that you are leaning away from your partner.

3 Bend sideways from the waist without leaning forward, as if you were standing between two sheets of glass. Don't let the space between your hips and ribs collapse. Hold this position for two breaths, then return to an upright position. As you breath out, slowly move your arm above your head and lean toward your partner.

4 *(left)* Stretch your outer arm slowly over toward your partner's until you are able to join hands, if possible. If this starts to hurt either person's back, just stretch your fingers toward each other without touching. Keep your waist long. Hold the stretch for a few breaths, and then repeat the stretch on the other side.

chest opener
exhilarating

open your chest and hips with these yoga postures

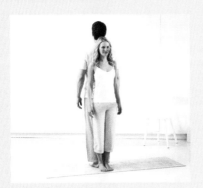

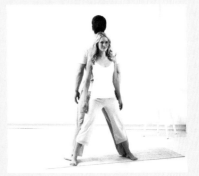

1 Remove your shoes and socks and stand back to back with your partner on a non-slip surface, such as a yoga mat. Press your back against your partner's back, or as close as your different heights will allow. Everything you do should be mirrored by your partner, so that you move as one. Tell each other at once if you need to stop.

2 Step your feet about a metre (3 feet) apart, or as far as feels safe. Hold your partner's hands if you wish: it may help you keep your balance. From here on, your partner should move left wherever you move right. Try to be sensitive to each other's balance and limitations. This is a good way of becoming more attuned to each other.

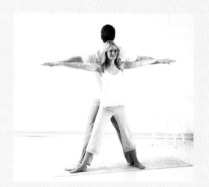
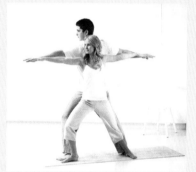

3 Turn your right foot out so your toes are pointing to the side. At the same time, your partner should turn their left foot to mirror yours. Turn your other foot inward slightly. Your hips and the rest of your body should remain facing forward throughout the exercise. Stretch your arms out to your sides, level with your shoulders.

4 Bend your right knee, without letting it go further forward than your toes, while your partner bends their left knee. You both should look toward the arm held above your bent knee. Keep your spine straight throughout. Check that your partner is comfortable. Hold this position for a few breaths, and then repeat it on the other side.

CHEST OPENER

1 Begin by standing separately. Stand with your feet hip-width apart, and take a step forward with your left foot. Raise your right hand in front of you about two palm-widths in front of your shoulders, palm facing forward. Bend your left knee slightly and move your weight onto your left foot. At the same time, extend your right palm further forward.

2 Breathe in and bring your weight backward onto your right foot. Lift the toes of your left foot as you do this. Bring your right arm back to a couple of palm-widths in front of your shoulders. Breathe in as you move backward and out as you move forward. Repeat this five times.

3 Move to face each other. Imagine a line on the floor between you. Both step forward to this line, so that your partner's left toes touch it on one side and your left toes touch it on the other side. Let your right palms touch: throughout this exercise, imagine you could hold a piece of paper between your palms without either crushing or dropping it.

4 *(right and opposite)* Move slowly forward while your partner moves backward. Breathe with the movement – one of you breathes out as the other breathes in. Don't let your knee bend further forward than your toes. Repeat with your right foot and left hand.

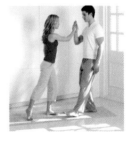

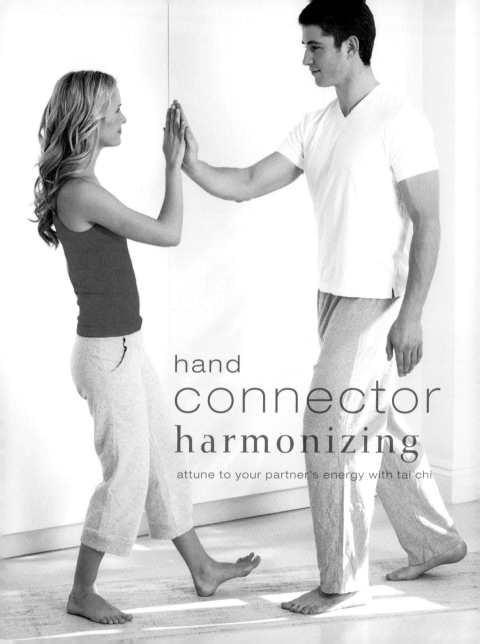

hand
connector
harmonizing

attune to your partner's energy with tai chi

1 Ask your partner to lie face down on a firm surface, such as on a towel on the floor. They can rest their forehead either on a cushion or on their folded arms. They don't need to take their clothes off for this massage, as the moves are all static. Kneel beside your partner.

2 Put the heels of your hands on each side of your partner's spine, starting near the base. Press into the muscles, avoiding the spine itself. Lift your hands and repeat, working your way up to their shoulders and outward across their upper back.

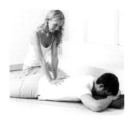

3 *(right)* Hold your partner's shoulders with your fingers in front and your thumbs behind. Using the pads of your thumbs, press into the muscles and make circles, feeling muscle move over bone rather than fingers over skin. Work around the edge of their shoulder blades with the same press-and-circle movement, and up the muscles of their neck.

4 Knead your partner's shoulder muscles with your hands – use the pads of your fingers rather than your fingertips. Work from the neck outward, and continue down their upper arms. Tell your partner to let you know if anything is uncomfortable – either if you're pressing too hard, or even not hard enough, which can tickle.

116

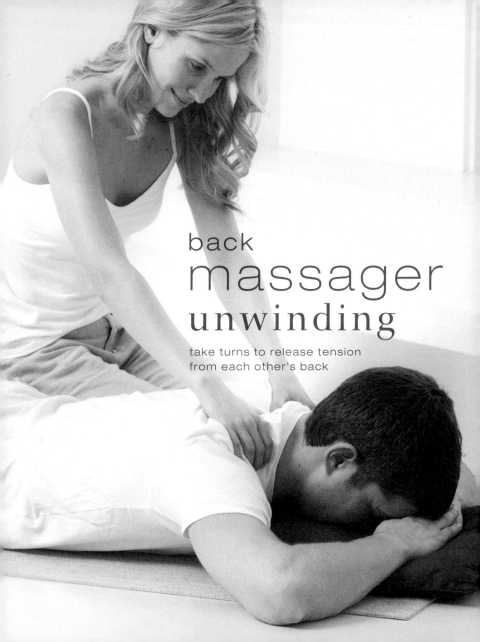

back massager
unwinding

take turns to release tension
from each other's back

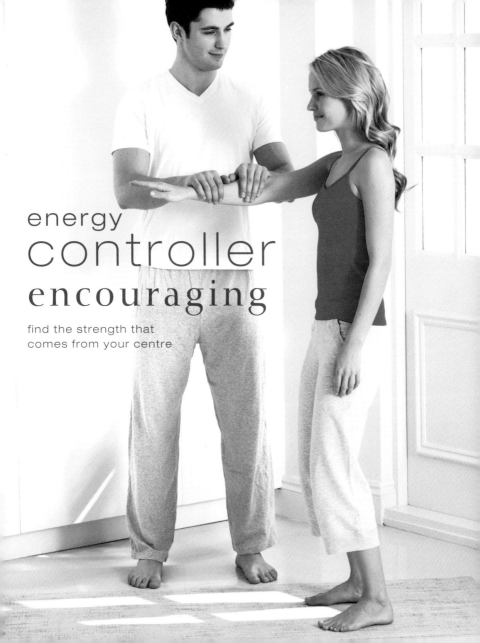

energy
controller
encouraging

find the strength that
comes from your centre

1

Stand with your feet a comfortable distance apart. Make sure your knees are soft – not bent, but not locked. Rock back and forth a couple of times and find the central point where you're not leaning forward or backward. Your back should be straight without being rigid, and your shoulders should be relaxed.

2

Close your eyes and let your breath slow down naturally. Imagine yourself breathing into the spot about three finger-widths below your navel (your hara), which is your body's energy centre. Fold your hands over this point and focus on centring yourself. (Your partner should not be doing the same yet.)

3

(left) Extend your right arm and invite your partner to try to push it up or down, either pressing your hand down or trying to bend your elbow. Try not to let your arm move, but don't resist with your muscles. Let your arm feel comfortable and stay focused on your hara, the source of your unshakeable inner strength.

4

Focus on something in the distance. Visualize the energy flowing from your hara along the length of your arm, filling it up like a hose filling with water. Imagine a torrent of energy pouring out through your hand. Your partner will probably be unable to move your arm. Then change places with your partner.

119

foot massager boosting

restore your energy with reflexology

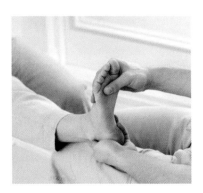

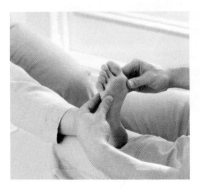

1 Rest your partner's right foot on your left knee. Cradle their foot in your left hand. Using firm but gentle pressure, rotate the ankle in both directions, then gently pull and rotate the toes. Using both hands, massage their whole foot with small circular motions, especially the sole. Your partner should tell you if anything is uncomfortable.

2 Holding their foot in both hands with your thumbs on the sole near the heel, slide your thumbs out to the sides. Move a short distance up the foot, repeat and continue – this should create a feeling of openness across the whole sole. Then bring your thumbs to the centre of the sole, just below the ball of the foot, and massage firmly.

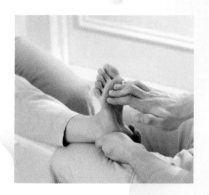

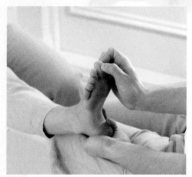

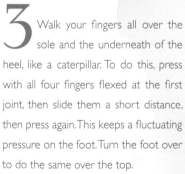

3 Walk your fingers all over the sole and the underneath of the heel, like a caterpillar. To do this, press with all four fingers flexed at the first joint, then slide them a short distance, then press again. This keeps a fluctuating pressure on the foot. Turn the foot over to do the same over the top.

4 Massage the big toe pad – press firmly into the centre with your thumb tip for 5 seconds, then do the same into the top of the toe, above the nail. Stroke firmly up the sides, from the ankle to the toes, and finish by briefly holding the foot in both hands. Repeat steps 1 to 4 on your partner's left foot.

121

1 Head massage is more relaxing when done by someone else, and avoids the risk of increasing tension in your own shoulders. Stand behind your partner, who is seated. Pour a few drops of almond oil into your hands and rub them together. Rub your fingertips briskly all over your partner's head as if you were lightly scratching it.

2 Stand beside your partner. Imagine a line running from their nose, up over their head. Press firmly beside this line with the tips of two fingers, starting between the eyebrows. Press in against the bone. Lift the pressure and repeat just above, continuing to the back of their head.

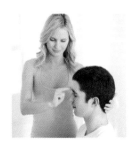

3 *(right)* Stand behind your partner and imagine lines running from each temple around the back of their head, and from the bottom of each ear diagonally back to their shoulders. Rub your fingertips up and down these lines using fairly firm pressure. Then, pressing your finger pads firmly into their scalp, massage all over it using a small circular motion.

4 Put your palms on the back of your partner's head, fingers pointing upward as if cupping the skull. Press upward, not pulling the hair but moving the scalp over the skull to release tension. Lift and move your hands to repeat around the edge of the hairline.

122

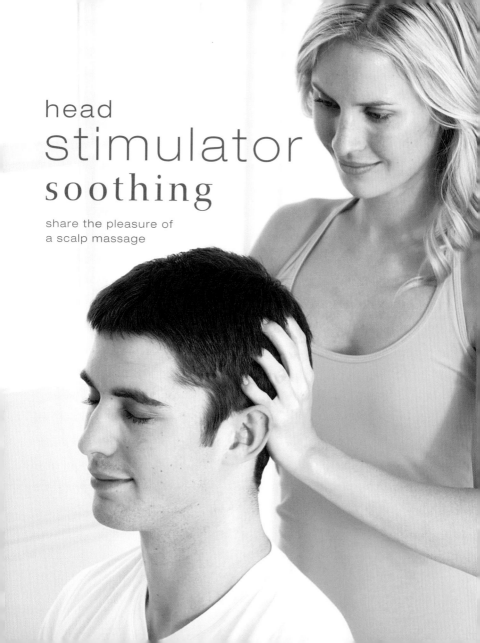

head
stimulator
soothing

share the pleasure of
a scalp massage

everyday sequences

If you are looking for a set of energizing exercises and have a little more time, use these menus to find what you need – reviving or refocusing, refreshing or simply energy-boosting. You can try these sequences in any suitable location.

half-hour reviver

38 sunday morning

56 on a plane

68 eye revitalizer

50 in your kitchen

64 scalp soother

70 throat releaser

half-hour refocuser

40 before a meeting

102 stress reliever

98 mental focuser

96 energy giver

90 mental refresher

94 strength restorer

half-hour lifter

92 vitality enhancer

60 at the park

40 before a meeting

76 leg invigorator

52 at your desk

30 afternoon wake-up

index

acknowledgments

author's acknowledgments

Janet Wright would like to thank everyone who has taught her, over many years, the techniques used in this book. Also Grace Cheetham, who created and oversaw the whole project; Katey Mackenzie, an inspired editor; and the photoshoot team – Jantje, Jules, Tinks, Adam, Tess and Joe – whose work so beautifully brings the ideas in this book to life. It's been a pleasure working with you all.

publisher's acknowledgments

Duncan Baird Publishers would like to thank models Tess Montgomery and Joe Griffith, hair and make-up artist Tinks Reding, photographer Jules Selmes and photographer's assistant Adam Giles.